INTENTIONAL HEALTH

*Your Best Chance for Aging Well
and Avoiding Chronic Health Conditions*

DR. GARY PETRO

This book is not intended to provide medical advice or take the place of medical advice and treatment from your personal physician. Readers are advised to consult their own doctors or other qualified health professionals regarding the treatment of their medical problems. Neither the publisher nor their author takes any responsibility for any possible consequences for any treatment, action, or application of medicine, supplement, herb, or preparation to any person reading or following the information in this book. If readers are taking prescription medications, they should consult with their physicians and not take themselves off any medicine without the proper supervision of a physician. To protect the privacy of the doctor's clients, stories recorded in this book are composite illustrations from the case histories of several individuals. All forms of exercise pose some inherent risk. The editors, publisher, and author advise readers to take full responsibility for their safety and know their limits before practicing any exercise. As with all exercise and dietary programs, you should get your doctor's approval before beginning.

GARY PETRO, D.C.

Printed in the United States of America
First Printing 2020
First Edition 2020

ISBN 978-1-7353401-0-4 paperback

10 9 8 7 6 5 4 3 2 1

Inquiries regarding permission for the use of material
contained in this book should be addressed to
Dr. Gary Petro
Good Medicine Functional Health
100 E. Second Street Suite #223
Whitefish, MT 59937
info@goodmedicinefh.com

This book is dedicated to Mary Claire, without whose support and inspiration this book would not have been written—she is my greatest encourager. And to my sons, who cared enough to give me that extra nudge to get over the finish line.

Contents

Forward

Today, at this very moment, our health and our life are the results of the choices we have made up to this point in time, like it or not. We may have made good choices or less than ideal choices; still, we remain today the accumulative effect of those choices. It is thus apparent, that the choices we make today will affect our future health and life.

Reading *Intentional Health* will give you the opportunity of a better future, by offering you more informed choices about your health. Allow me to explain:

Let's say you're driving down the road and your check engine light comes on. An indication, a symptom, if you will, that something might be wrong with the vehicle you are driving. You have choices! You can see the check engine light is on, but you could choose to ignore it. You can see that the check engine light is on and cover it up with some tape, so you don't see it anymore, essentially ignoring that there is a potential problem. Another option would be to stop at a facility where an educated individual concerning the functioning of an automobile, could thoroughly evaluate as to why the check engine light is on and after the comprehensive examination attempt to fix the problem. Whether you ignore the problem or fix the problem-each is still a choice with future consequences. The same holds true with your health!

What you will need to do will be explained in a very understandable manner. You will see that Dr. Petro's approach to helping someone with improving their health and life is by providing a way to navigate and sort through health information based on a new way of thinking about health and disease. He wants to find the right treatment for each person, regardless of what the treatment might be. If pharmacology is the best treatment, he may recommend that; if a change in diet, nutraceutical supplements, or lifestyle change works best, then he will choose that. Dr. Petro's fundamental approach is that he has chosen to treat the person, not the disease, the system, not just the symptoms. This is truly personalized medicine, the healthcare practice of the future. This type of care is considered Functional Medicine--a new way to understand the underlying causes of disease in how our genes, our environment, and our lifestyle interact to determine our own health and/or disease.

You will find that Dr. Petro wants to answer the question "Why?"-- Not just, "What is the right drug or supplement for this disease?" The question also is not, "What disease do you have?" but "Which system or systems in your body are out of balance?" The goal is to understand what disturbs the normal function of the systems, and how we can best create optimal function. Essentially, he treats the whole YOU! This is the methodology of care that "just makes sense!" I have known Dr. Petro for over 30 years. He exemplifies an individual who has dedicated his life through a great deal of self-discipline in educating himself on cutting edge technology and practice management to provide the best possible care to his patients. You will not be disappointed.

I commend you, the reader, on making the right choice of enhancing your future health through Functional Medicine. Enjoy the process of discovery of the new you!

Dr. James R. Grilliot
Chiropractic Physician

Introduction

When I am asked, "What kind of patients do you treat?" my answer is quite simple. I treat *frustrated* patients. These are people who want to feel great but, due to choices, circumstances, and their continued symptoms, who have lost hope. Frustrated patients have a real dilemma. They have had at least one significant health-related problem for an extended period--many times for years. Initially, they focused on their symptoms and tried relieving them using different methods. Many people first search the web for home treatment ideas and then visit their physician, who often refers them to a specialist. After many tests, significant costs, and much time, their condition is often more severe than when it all began. There comes a time when the original symptoms become secondary to the frustration these patients feel, often leading to anger, depression, or anxiety.

I grew up in a household that was not overly concerned about health. Looking back, we ate the Standard American Diet (SAD) with the vegetables limited to peas, corn, and lima beans, which are mostly starch. I was very overweight in my childhood and teen years. Due to my weight in elementary and middle school, I was called names and often picked in the last rounds for any type of athletic team. I started playing tennis in high school and won most of my matches not because I could get around the court fast—I couldn't—but because it was difficult for my opponents to return my serve. It is amazing how we adapt to situations. I had always wanted to be a veterinarian, so I went to Michigan State University but during those four years so much changed. My focus shifted to engineering. Then I met the girl of my dreams, fell in love, and got married. During this same time, my outlook on life changed dramatically. I had been an atheist, with no room for spirituality. Science would solve the world's issues. I even thought that I would have my body frozen in a cryogenic tank in hopes that future medical technology might be able to someday revive and restore my body to full health. I saw life as finite.

God, however, had a different direction for me. My conversion to Christianity was not my plan but God's. As I started my spiritual journey, I thought my faith would be in constant conflict with science, but it wasn't. The world is much more complex than can be explained by science alone. When I consider the human body, I see the intricate detail of the millions of chemical reactions occurring every second that allow our bodies to keep functioning. The ability of the body to adapt and change to the environment is the cornerstone of why I do what I do. I have seen the power of God's healing by miraculously removing tumors, healing open skin lesions in a fraction of normal healing time, and restoring cognitive function when there were no medical explanations. My faith affects every area of my life. I believe God has given each of us a body to take care of properly; we only get one.

By applying good lifestyle skills (diet, sleep, exercise, and stress control) along with proper testing and follow-through, you can see a metamorphosis of your health. It is never too late to start your journey to better health, but it does take intentionality. My passion is to help you regain your health and for you to say, "I never thought I could feel so good."

I have 35 years of clinical practice, with the last 22 years devoted to Functional Medicine, clinical nutrition, and utilizing both standard and functional testing to solve the puzzles of chronic illness. In my practice, I have seen patients of all ages, from infants a few days old to those in their eighties with chronic health conditions. For many patients with chronic health conditions, a typical consultation with their physician or specialist might go like this: "All of your tests have come back, and I have reviewed them. I can't find anything wrong with you." Then it goes downhill, with comments like, "Maybe it will go away," "You know, you *are* getting older," or "How about I write a prescription for an antidepressant to help you?" If you are like most frustrated patients, at this point, you want to scream. I am here to tell you that every person can find a step-by-step path to recover their health. That is what this book will assist you to do.

This book is not for you if:

- You think our current health care system can and will meet all your health needs.
- You are in excellent health, able to do all the activities that you want.

- You do not care about potential diseases later in life.
- You are living a full life, sleep great, and feel peace throughout the day.

If that is your situation, I congratulate you—keep it up! I encourage you to give this book to someone you know who is struggling with their health.

This book <u>is for you</u> if:

- You are not satisfied with your current health and the health care system.
- You believe there is more to life than you are currently experiencing.
- You believe you can feel much better but do not know what to do, or where to begin.

You are the type of person who is willing to invest your time and resources to make it happen. Just remember: hope is not a strategy.

Ultimately, your health decisions are yours and yours alone. Don't relegate your health to others. As much as they might care for you, ultimately, you are the one that must live with your symptoms, conditions, and your choices. I hope that, by the time you finish reading this book, you will have a better understanding of how you can take control of your body to repair, regenerate, and heal.

Chapter One

How Did I Get Here?

"In order to change, we must be sick and tired
of being sick and tired."
~ Unknown

The Disease Model and a Health Care Crisis

We are in a health care crisis in this country. A 2019 Gallup poll found that 70% of the U.S. population believes our health care system has a "major problem" or is in a "state of crisis" and has been that way for many years.[1] Compared to ten other countries—the U.K., Canada, Germany, Australia, Japan, Sweden, France, Denmark, the Netherlands, and Switzerland—U.S. life expectancy was the lowest. Infant mortalities were the highest.[2] In the U.S., we spend nearly 20% of our GDP on health care--almost twice as much as any other country--yet we still score poorly compared to other countries' population health. There are so many excuses presented, and unfortunately, many are political. *If* we expect to change these poor statistics, it is going to take personal responsibility. That is why this book is called *Intentional Health*. You need to be responsible for yourself and, if you have children, their health as well. Gone are the days that you can blindly just do what the organized health system tells you to do. We keep building bigger and more hospitals while, at the same time, our world is becoming less healthy. Right now, we are all under COVID-19 mandates. What is interesting is that most of the recommendations and mandates are not based on scientific data, but on opinion and delaying the course of the virus.

I believe most people genuinely want to feel energetic, enjoy life, sleep well, and take minimal medication if any. We have been in a disease-based model of health care for many years because of insurance companies taking over health care. This has placed attention on a person's symptoms and the goal of just getting the symptoms stabilized. This model has failed miserably. In addition, the insurance industry's control of health care means that patients have been time-shorted by doctors for many years. One reason for this time-shorting recently came to light in an article in the *Journal of General Internal Medicine*.[3] The article studied randomly selected patients at the Mayo Clinic and affiliated clinics in Minnesota and Wisconsin. In most of the encounters (64% of the primary physicians and 80% of the specialists), the doctor did not even question the patient about why they were there. When the doctor did allow the patient to explain the reason for their visit, most of the doctors interrupted quickly, at an average of 11 seconds.

Even if your experience is much better than this alarming statistic, one must admit doctor/patient interaction time for most patients has decreased significantly over the past few decades. In the disease-based model of care, the most important thing is the symptom and how to best hide or control it. This becomes a ticking time bomb because the symptoms will become progressively worse. Many times, people find their doctor increasing the dosage of the medication because their body has adapted, now requiring a larger dose to have the same effect. Delay in identification and treatment of the root problems only leads to increased stress, frustration, and lost productivity. We should instead be using a model that understands symptoms are important, but even more important is the cause of the symptoms.

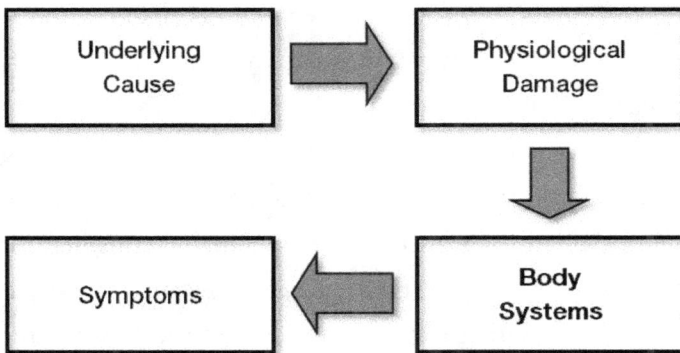

```
┌──────────────┐        ┌──────────────┐
│  Underlying  │   ⟹   │ Physiological│
│    Cause     │        │    Damage    │
└──────────────┘        └──────────────┘
                               ⇓
┌──────────────┐        ┌──────────────┐
│              │   ⟸   │     Body     │
│   Symptoms   │        │   Systems    │
└──────────────┘        └──────────────┘
```

Many patients have disclosed in their consultation that they have been told it is "all in their heads." Granted, some people do have severe emotional issues that bring on symptoms that can mimic true physiological problems, but this is not often the case in my practice. Normally, it is the opposite: their underlying physiological issues bring about the emotional dysfunction due to neurotransmitter imbalances because of gut dysfunction, adrenal imbalances, or hormonal issues. With proper amino acid treatment, even these emotional problems can be resolved in a natural way. Anti-depressants have become one of the most prescribed medications for off-label use when the standard medication does not resolve the patient's symptoms. Anti-depressant use rose by 65% between 1999 and 2014, with one in eight Americans over the age of 12 using them. The only way we can have true healing is to understand the root problems.

Great health does not just happen. It is a process of small steps, each working towards the larger goal. It takes personal responsibility to decide to change.

Do you ever dream about what your life would be like if you didn't have that pain that prevents you from playing with your kids or grandkids, that digestive issue that keeps you from traveling very far from home, that skin condition that you always wear clothing to cover? I could tell you story after story that would break your heart from the thousands of patients I have seen. During consultations, I often ask my patients to share their stories so I can hear why they finally decided to do something about their health. Too often it is not that they have not done anything. Rather, what they have done has not helped, and they were never given plan B. Rarely were they ever recommended to change their lifestyle with diet, exercise, brain activities, or emotional work. This frustration has caused them to lose hope that they can return to optimal health. The sad reality is, most people see little change, not because they are not trying, but because they aren't finding the right starting point to turn their condition around. They expect the same old routines to provide a different result than they have previously experienced.

FUNCTIONAL MEDICINE: A PATIENT-CENTERED APPROACH

As opposed to the disease-based model described above, I believe a patient-centered approach, which looks at the whole person and what has led to their symptoms, is the best way to find the underlying dysfunction. I like to think of it as an onion. If you cut the onion in half, crosswise, there will be many concentric rings. The core represents a patient's root problem--how it originally began. The rings represent the different symptoms (or health conditions) that have evolved because of the core issue and adaptation. Remember the popular definition of insanity? It's doing the same thing repeatedly, expecting a different result. The goal of this book is to help you understand better how to get to the core of your onion. For most people, there is great hope to turn around your health and get your life back.

Although Functional Medicine is becoming more known and understood, patients have not been made aware that Functional Medicine can revolutionize their health. Listening to a patient's story can give a great insight into the significant event(s) that have led to his or her current state of ill-health. This process takes time. In my practice, a consultation with a new patient with a chronic condition takes an hour to an hour and a half. That is how long it takes to cover their history properly, even after reading the twenty-some pages of information that they complete before the consultation. Appropriate tests with the proper interpretation, as well as a thorough functional exam are the gold standard for giving insight and clarity to what appears to be the core problem(s). It is this understanding that can give hope for a better, more energized, and fulfilling life.

A described above, one of the biggest difficulties with our health care system today is the focus on symptoms and not taking the time to delve into the actual problems. This is where Functional Medicine shines. It is a biological approach to identifying and treating the root causes of disease. For example, a person's elevated cholesterol issue could be the result of a heart problem, liver problem, blood sugar problem, digestive problem, genetic issue, etc. There might not even be a problem with the elevated cholesterol if the inflammation markers, hormone levels, and blood viscosity tests are normal. Yes, that's right. A person with elevated cholesterol can have a *lower* risk of cardiovascular accidents than a person with normal or low cholesterol.

Let's consider an iceberg. It is both beautiful and dangerous at the same time. What we see on top of the water is beautiful with the crisp white, blue, and sometimes green colors of the rugged spires and cliffs. What lays under the water is the remaining seven-eighths of the iceberg. This is the mass that holds the iceberg from tipping over in the rough seas. This is also the part that has taken many large transoceanic vessels out. The portion on top of the water represents a person's symptoms, or, what they feel--the pain, brain fog, abnormal bowel movements, difficulty losing weight, thyroid issues, fatigue, etc. This is often the only portion addressed by most physicians in our current health care system. The seven-eighths under water signify what has happened in a patient's life, which has led up to the health problems. It includes previous treatment or lack of treatment, eating habits, stress situations, lack of or over-exercise, sleep habits, genetics, and other factors. These conditions and choices over time have allowed the portion above the water to become more visible as time progresses. If there wasn't a base to the iceberg, there would not be the visible top. As the base (underlying physiologic dysfunction) is melted, the visible portion (patients' symptoms) decreases in size until both disappear.

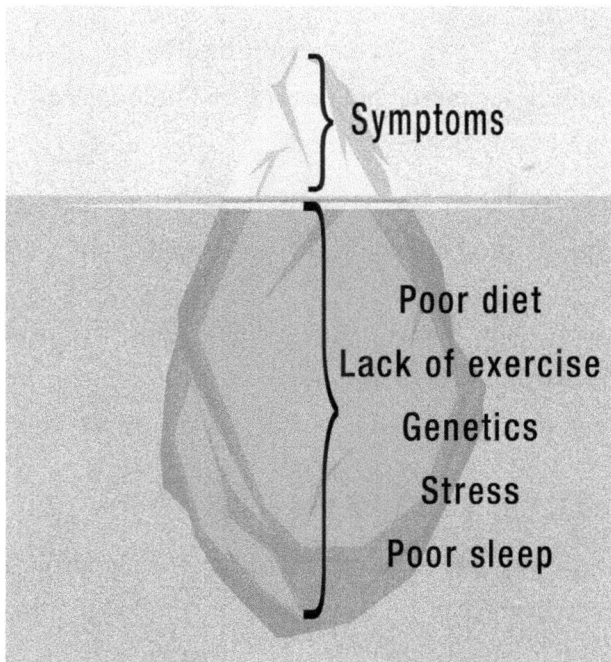

~ 15 ~

OPTIMAL HEALTH FUNDAMENTALS

1. Most people want to have great health. To accomplish this, accountability is essential.

2. Health is a journey. Some changes happen quickly, and other underlying problems can take years to resolve.

3. Great health is comprised of nutritional, physical, emotional, and genetic factors.

4. Once you start on a path to better health, there will be situations that work at derailing the process. It is up to each of us to get back on the path.

5. If you choose to improve your health, you need to do it for yourself. Changing habits for loved ones never leads to long-term change.

6. People who choose to make the necessary changes will enjoy a greater level of health, joy, and happiness.

Let me explain how Functional Medicine and the Optimal Health Fundamentals apply to real patient scenarios, using two patients with chronic problems, with two different outcomes, as an example.

THE TALE OF TWO PATIENTS

As a rule, the younger a person is the faster they respond. A child, even only a few months old treated for colic or other digestive conditions will usually show improvement in a matter of days to weeks compared to a person in their 60's with comorbidities that can take 3-6 months to see any progress. Many older people believe it is too late to revitalize their health. The truth is: if you want better health, you can get it. If you don't want to take responsibility for your health, you will stay where you are and most likely become progressively worse. When I think of patients that had an opportunity to become a better version of themselves, two come to mind. Here are their stories. (I have changed names and certain details to protect privacy.)

CASE STUDY: JOHN

John (not his real name) came in for recurrent back pain. I had treated John many years earlier for a similar problem and he did well until this recent flareup. Before retirement, John worked in accounting for a larger corporation. He has been retired for several years and keeps himself moderately busy with minimal physical activity. After his recent back pain was under control, we talked about other health issues. He shared that he has been plagued for the last 20 years with chronic digestive issues. He had to be incredibly careful where he went and how long it would take to get there because of unpredictable diarrhea. He was only able to travel for less than 30 minutes without being concerned about his digestive issues. Also, he suffered from depression, diabetes, thyroid dysfunction, prostate hypertrophy, high cholesterol, and gout, in addition to fatigue. His current medication (with potential side effects listed in brackets) included:

- Two different blood sugar regulators {complications leading to amputations, diabetic acidosis, kidney injury, vitamin B12 deficiency, vomiting, sleepiness, muscle pain, fever, or chills, diarrhea, and flatulence}

- A statin drug for high cholesterol {constipation, diarrhea, nausea, fatigue, gas, heartburn, headache, and muscle pain}

- Levothyroxine for decreased thyroid function {chest pain/shortness of breath, irritability, sleeplessness, diarrhea, muscle cramps, headache, hair loss, tremors, nervousness, and inability to tolerate heat}

- Tamsulosin for prostate issues {painful or difficult–urination, lower back and flank pain, chest pain, and dizziness}

- Allopurinol to reduce the production of uric acid that causes gout {drowsiness, headache, diarrhea, gastric pain, altered taste, bruising, and muscle pain}

- Tylenol PM for sleep and muscle achiness

- Levomefolate calcium

With all this in mind, I wanted to delve into finding John's core health issues. I ordered the necessary tests (only a short panel because he'd had a blood test a few months earlier and it wasn't necessary to re-run them all). Within a few weeks, we sat down to discuss the results. The food sensitivity test results indicated changes in diet were necessary. Based on a reading of his blood test using Functional Medicine optimal values, there were some significant results indicating not just a thyroid problem, but autoimmune thyroiditis, also known as Hashimoto's disease. His fasting blood glucose was 135 even with his medications. Kidneys were showing signs of stress. Liver enzymes elevated, low vitamin D, and low magnesium. One of the extremely good signs was the absence of inflammation markers in his blood. An adrenal stress profile was run and showed that he was struggling in the morning to get going. The test looks at 4-time intervals during the day, (morning, within 30 minutes after waking; noon; around 4 pm; and then again before bedtime). The morning level was significantly lower than the recommended values, indicating a progressing adrenal issue. The last test I ran on John was a DNA stool sample. The results were as expected. He still had C. Diff of both toxins A & B, four strains of dysbiosis bacteria overgrowth, Candida (yeast), a parasite, and significant inflammation within the colon.

At this point, we had enough information to develop a protocol for John. This was the plan:

- John would need to restrict gluten, eggs, dairy, certain nuts, and dietary yeast.

- Due to the overlapping chronic problems, I started him on adaptogenic herbs and morning licorice root drops.

- Vitamin D3 A high EPA/DHA Omega 3.

- For the significant bowel issues, I used a multi-botanical to target the entire digestive tract along with

Saccharomyces Boulardii during the day and a multi-strain probiotic before bed to help repair and restore at night.

- The last supplement was a magnesium L-Threonate. I chose this form of magnesium due to his age and memory decline. He did not have a serious decline but was forgetting more than he thought was acceptable.

Normally, I would address the adrenal issue first but because only the morning cortisone level was elevated, I elected to move right into the digestive treatment.

During the consultation, John and I spent sufficient time reviewing the test and why he needed to do both the dietary restriction and supplementation and make lifestyle changes. I counseled him that once he started having more energy, exercises would be increased but for now, walking would be appropriate. John was agreeable and I scheduled to see him back in a few weeks to help monitor his progress.

When I saw John again, I was not so encouraged. He was having a hard time complying with his dietary restrictions. He was getting most of his supplements in, but he and his wife traveled most workdays during the day to help a young relative. They left early in the morning, stopping for a donut or a fast-food breakfast. For lunch, they would go out to grab something, mainly at fast-food restaurants. Then, they would eat dinner out on their way home. On the weekends, John worked at eating more in line with the recommendations I had given him. I understood John's issue struggling to find appropriate food to eat where they were. I tried to explain again the importance of making the harder choice to plan for his eating. I suggested planning the night before for his breakfast with easy choices. Lunch could be brought in a cooler to ensure he would be getting the high-quality nutrition that was necessary for his body to heal optimally. For dinner, a possibility would be to use their oven or crockpot automated cycle so the food would be done around the time they arrived home. Then it would only take a short time to fix a few nutritious side dishes. The other issue was that John's wife was not on board. Since she did not have digestive problems like John, she was not as supportive as she might have been, which would have been a valuable help for John. Nevertheless, he agreed to work at making the changes.

I saw him again in about a month. He felt that making the changes was too difficult and did not think he could do it. He was still having a donut and coffee for breakfast, eating out at fast food sub shops or pizza for lunch, and a local restaurant for most evening meals. The benefit and hope of having normal bowel movements, normalized blood sugar, and more energy was not as great as the effort he needed to change. Once again, we discussed making modifications, but John did not think he could follow the recommendations. To be honest, I was frustrated. Here was a genuinely nice gentleman who suffered multiple significant chronic health problems which caused a substantial decrease in his quality of life. If only he would take responsibility for his daily health choices, he had a high probability of significantly improving his life. I do not think John could see himself ever living without his chronic health issues.

CASE STUDY: JANE

Jane (not her real name) came to our practice with complaints of constant left leg pain with difficulty walking, low back pain, chronic fatigue, food intolerance, difficulty swallowing, multiple joint pain, overweight, headaches, digestive issues, couldn't sleep through the night, and pulmonary fibrosis. She was under the care of a pulmonologist at a leading university hospital. She had also been under the care of an orthopedist and chiropractor. She was old enough to retire but was finishing out one more year in the HR/accounting department of a local manufacturing plant. She was a very pleasant person who was able to explain her complaints clearly.

On examination, Jane was found to be deconditioned with marked muscle weakness, had an inflamed tender abdomen, and muscle tenderness. Also, there was difficulty with balance, elevated blood pressure, and bilateral knee positive orthopedic tests. Like many patients, she was already on multiple nutritional supplements, without the improvement for which she had hoped. I ran a thorough blood panel looking at a wide range of body systems, plus organic acid, and food sensitivity tests.

The results showed that she had systemic inflammation.

- Two blood test markers I use are ESR, and CRP-hs levels. The CRP-hs should be less than .5 mg/dL for optimal level and the ESR less than 10 mm/hr. Jane's CR-hs was 18.9 mg/dL (almost 40 times the upper level), and her ESR at 57

- Magnesium was low

- Vitamin D was 28 with optimal ranging between 50-90

- She had serious iron deficiency

- Liver not clearing well

- A high uric acid marker for gout

- Blood sugar only a few points from the diabetic level

- Her urine pH was very acidic

- Other markers were less significant but still out of the optimal range

- Her organic acid test revealed fatty acid metabolism problems, neuroendocrine dysfunction, oxidative damage, bacterial and yeast infiltration of her gut.

Clearly, the multi-layering of problems required planning to address both her current symptoms as well as to treat the underlying problems that led to the symptoms. Our priority was getting the inflammation down first and start to up-regulate her iron levels. The plan we discussed was over time, to:

- Implement a modified ketogenic diet to help with reducing the inflammation, and supplement with curcumin

- Take Bis-Glycinate Chelate iron for her severely low iron level

- Address the GI issues with a multiherbal to kill off the unwanted pathogens, enzymes with HCL to improve digestion, and probiotics for the re-establishment of gut flora

- Magnesium and potassium for pH balance

- Liposomal glutathione and Vitamin C for detoxification and antioxidation

Over six months, Jane made an excellent improvement. About two months after starting the initial protocol, her iron levels were in the optimal range, her Systolic Blood pressure was now averaging in the 120s. Her most significant change was with her CRP-hs inflammation marker, which was down to less than one. She lost 20 pounds, was sleeping through the night, and her leg pain was almost gone. She said she was now able to load the dishwasher with no pain!

I made interim changes to the program based on the repeat tests and Jane felt like she was getting her life back. She continued through the rest of the program, and with the reduction of inflammation, she was able to start building her body up. This resulted in the ability to go on walks, and her brain fog was gone. Her pulmonologist was thrilled with her progress. Most importantly, Jane was becoming a better version of herself.

Several months after she started having the positive changes in her healing, I asked why she was willing to put the time into her program with the modified eating, taking the prescribed supplements, exercise, and lifestyle changes. She explained that she would be retiring soon, had a lot she wanted to do after retirement, and knew she would not be able to do those things the way she was feeling before.

Jane held tightly to her life goals that helped keep her on the plan to achieve her successes, whereas John was only looking day-to-day without being able to see how the benefits would change his life. So, as you can see, your outlook and life goals are integral to your healing. You are the only one that can decide to change.

CHILDREN ARE NOT IMMUNE

I am grateful for the advancement in acute emergency medicine, new surgical procedures, and diagnostic testing. The problem is that most health problems fall into the category of chronic health conditions. Chronic conditions are generally understood as being present for at least three months or longer and often progress down a path of increasing intensity and/or disability. 80% of the people in the United States age 65 and older have one chronic condition, and 77% have two or more.[4] We can understand some of that due to increasing age, however, a whopping 25% of children under age five have at least one chronic condition.[5] These children are starting to go through life with a significant disadvantage.

I have seen a constant stream of infants for failure to thrive and digestive problems in the first three months of life. Most of the time, before my seeing these babies, the main treatment has been medication with little or no improvement. The baby cries excessively and gets little sleep, or the baby is lethargic. The parents cannot sleep, and the irritability and frustration factor rises exponentially in the whole family. My heart breaks for families going through this. Usually, they leave my consultation with hope by understanding how failure to thrive happens. The first thing we do is listen carefully to the parent as they explain the timeline of the baby's condition. If the mom is breastfeeding, it is common for her to transfer reactive proteins to the baby through her breastmilk. If the baby is not receiving breast milk, the formula he or she is ingesting has food or additives that are most often causing the inflammation and irritation to the baby's digestive tract. Treatment can be quite simple at that point: making sure the baby is not ingesting the foods that cause irritation and upregulating the baby's immune system. It is such a joy to hear during a follow-up visit that the parents and the baby are getting the sleep they need, the baby is not spitting up excessively, and peace has come back to the family.

Treating children with the Functional Medicine approach is no different than treating adults. The goal is always to determine the underlying issue for the symptom. If infants and children are not able to digest and process the food they eat, improper absorption will occur. It is in the digestive tract that all the vitamins and minerals are absorbed into the blood. Improper absorption of nutrients can cause learning disabilities (Autism, Spectrum Disorders, etc.), chronic digestive problems, emotional issues, and more.

Think of proper food as gas for your car. I was once traveling to another state for a meeting. I left early in the morning and near a major city, stopped for gas. I filled up and got back on the highway. Within a minute, blue smoke started pouring out of the tailpipe and the car sputtered and died. After having it towed to two different repair shops with no idea what was going on, a wise older mechanic asked if they had checked the fuel in the tank. They found there was diesel fuel in a gasoline tank. They drained the diesel, put gasoline in, and I was on my way. The next day I contacted the gas station, and they said the underground tank was mistakenly filled with diesel instead of gasoline. Here's the correlation: Our bodies, whether we are a child or an adult, need to run on the right gas (diet) to function properly. There is no one-size-fits-all diet.

DROWNING IN HEALTH INFORMATION

We are in an age of information overload. You can find just about anything related to health on the Internet and still there is a great struggle for good health. A person scouring the web looking for information on type 2 diabetes will find an overabundance of ideas, products, and diets—some good, some off-the-wall, and many based on old data that continues to be rehashed. The other problem concerning health care information overload is contradictory research. One article might say that you should do a keto diet and another article the next week indicates that a keto diet can cause harm. So, which is it? Both are right. For some people, a keto diet plan can be beneficial, and for others, it is not helpful. We are all genetically different and what works for one might not be the best for another.

The question is What do *you* need? There is a multitude of excellent research happening in the health sciences regarding diseases and conditions, with new reports being published almost daily. PubMed is a free resource supporting the search and retrieval of peer-reviewed biomedical and life sciences literature to improve health–both globally and personally. The information is housed at the U.S. National Library of Medicine and is under the Department of Health and Human Services. In 2017 alone, they added almost 900,000 citations and abstracts. This comes down to about 1.7 papers filed every minute of every day. I am grateful that this information is available, however, the published results must be evaluated based on the type of study, the population base, and protocol. I spend many hours each week reviewing current studies and am constantly modifying my treatment procedures because of good, well-designed research.

Helping patients heal is a constantly evolving discipline that I love. Unfortunately, much of this current information will take many years to filter down to regular patient care in a disease-based healthcare model focused on symptom care rather than the underlying cause(s).

The PSA test is an example of research being incorrectly applied within the health care system. In 1970, Richard J. Ablin, Ph.D., DSc (Hon), first discovered the prostate-specific antigen (PSA) test for men. At the time, he and his associates were trying to identify a specific antigen for prostate cancer. Instead, they identified a PSA that is present not only in malignant prostates but also in non-cancerous prostates. To Alvin's dismay, more than two decades later, the U.S. FDA approved the test not only for the *recurrence* of prostate cancer but also as a possible *predictor* of prostate cancer. According to Dr. Alvin, it was fear and money that was being generated by the screenings, not health care outcomes. He went on to state the Schering-Plough Pick gave 1.2 million dollars to an American firm to promote PSA screening. Primary care physicians were brainwashed into thinking that, if they did not do a PSA test and a male patient subsequently was diagnosed with prostate cancer, the doctor could be sued. Dr. Alvin said there was a real misconception that lives are being saved with this test, which simply wasn't the case. In 2014, Dr. Alvin stated that the U.S. health care system is broken.[6] Unfortunately, many physicians are still using this mostly useless test.

SUPPLEMENTS: A CAUTIONARY TALE

The natural healthcare arena is no better and often worse in terms of applying research properly. Besides the multitude of drug stores, grocery stores, department stores, big-box stores, cosmetic stores, gas stations, etc., we have numerous multi-level "nutrition" companies. These multi-level companies are particularly confusing to consumers. Most of the sales come from regular people selling to their friends, work associates, family, and others. They have sales brochures stating what symptoms a particular product can be used for, without the understanding of the multitude of factors regarding proper use. I am sure many of these people are passionate about wanting to help but most lack training in even the most basic physiology and biochemistry. I do understand that people have been helped with their symptoms, but the real question is, have the underlying conditions improved? If the underlying cause is not changed, I see little difference between covering a symptom with a supplement rather than a drug. The only benefit is the side effects are minimal or nonexistent.

Another key caution regarding nutritional supplements is quality. In the U.S., there are three levels of supplementation:

- Pharmaceutical grade: This offers the highest quality and meets pharmaceutical standards.

- Food grade (store grade): These include ingredients that are suitable enough for people to eat. They do not have a rigorous screening process for the component ingredients or the final product.

- Feed grade (agricultural grade): These include ingredients suitable to feed animals and is also the lowest grade of supplements offered in the U.S.

Often, store grade supplementation uses cheaper raw products. For example, many of the minerals are oxide, which is much less bioavailable than the better brands that use chelated minerals for easier absorption. Sometimes, it doesn't matter; most of the time, it does.

We all understand that everyone wants to make wise use of their money. However, in many cases, the cheaper retail store brands, and multi-levels brands (food grade) are much more expensive in the long run. For example, one of my patients brought in a food-grade probiotic they were using. We compared the ingredients and colony count with a pharmaceutical-grade bottle. Even though her bottle was less expensive than the pharmaceutical-grade bottle, when we factored in the colony count strength, it would have taken 50 bottles to equal the potency of the one bottle that was only slightly more expensive.

In 2015, investigators tested several top-selling brands of medicinal herbs at national retailers, including GNC, Target, Walgreens, and Walmart. "The tests showed that pills labeled medicinal herbs often contained little more than cheap fillers like powdered rice, asparagus and houseplants, and in some cases substances that could be dangerous to those with allergies."[7] At some of the retailers, they found that 80% of other products tested did not contain any of the herbs on the labels. One of the store brands at Walgreens, a ginseng product that promoted "physical endurance and vitality," only contained powdered garlic and rice. At Walmart, a Ginkgo Biloba product promoted as a memory enhancer contained primarily powder radish, house plants, and wheat, even though it claimed to be gluten-free. We really shouldn't be surprised by this because, as the demand for health supplements increases, the bottom line is for some manufacturers the all-important factor. This is one of the reasons many people take supplements without seeing any benefit. I do not believe supplements should be regulated by governmental oversight, but I do recommend that you only take high-quality supplements. Like most industries, there will always be companies that want to take advantage of consumers.

If you are taking supplements for a while and not seeing the changes for which you were hoping, it could be due to several reasons:

- A variation in your genome could be inhibiting proper chemical synthesis of certain vitamins, minerals, and/or nutrients in your body
- The product you are taking is of poor quality, without enough of the active ingredients in the tablet or capsule
- Potency is not at therapeutic levels

Responsible supplement manufacturers have extensive quality control measures. Check the quality of the raw materials as well as the finished product. Many higher quality brands are not sold directly to the public.

Often, our population is looking for the latest greatest new supplement instead of looking at a whole health approach. I call it "the Roulette approach." Just look at the checkout counters of most stores. You will find magazines touting that "This supplement will make you into a new person!"—of course, with a photoshopped "before" and "after" picture. The Council for Responsible Nutrition (CRN) published data this year that showed about 77% of U.S.

adults take at least one dietary supplement in 2019 as compared to 65% in 2009. In the 18 to 34-years age group, approximately 70% take dietary supplements. And 79% in the over 55 age group take dietary supplements. Males and females are pretty much equally divided, as well as regions of the country.[8] It's more important than ever that patients are informed about effective supplement use and that a Functional Medicine approach is taken to ensure supplement use is not simply masking symptoms.

THE TREND TO NATURAL HEALTH

There has been a lot of doom and gloom covered in this chapter. However, even though the state of the nation's health is poor and there are many problems with the health care system, I am optimistic. Every month I see more and more articles—both in the professional journals and consumer magazines—encouraging a change to a more natural lifestyle. I feel fortunate to be at the forefront of these initiatives that will revolutionize our healthcare system. The momentum has been building over the past 40 years and we are at a tipping point. The drug companies want healthcare to remain status quo, but this tsunami of natural health and Functional Medicine will overtake the status quo. Then we will see a significant reduction in disease and increased longevity.

You can start this right here, right now, with your health. In the next chapter, we will explore the Functional Health Index (FHI). This is a guide that can help you determine if you need to be concerned about your current state of health.

Key Takeaways

- Having great health is about my daily choices.

- Poor health does not happen overnight; the problems start before there are symptoms.

- It is never too late to begin my health transformation.

- The vast amount of healthcare information confuses rather than helps most people.

- There is no one-size-fits-all plan.

- Using supplements to cover symptoms is little better than covering symptoms with medication.

Chapter Two

What's Your FHI?

Those who think they have no time for health prevention will sooner or later have to find time for illness.

A few months ago, an ax-throwing business opened near me. I have never thrown an ax inside, so I went along with a couple of my sons to try it out. Inside the ax-throwing center, there are lanes about 8 feet wide, separated with chain link fence from the floor to ceiling. About 15 feet away from the throwing line is a wood panel with a red bullseye. And, like most games using a bullseye, the closer you get to the center, the more points you get. We were shown how to throw an ax properly. They made it look so easy! As you can expect, the learning curve was a little steep. After about 30 throws, I started to get the hang of it and had a good time. It's not necessarily how hard the ax is thrown, but the technique that makes the difference.

The bullseye is a great way to visualize our health, with the center of the bullseye being optimal health. As we move to the outer circles, our health declines.

In this chapter, we are going to be looking at a tool I have created, the Functional Health Index (FHI) to determine where your health is in relationship to the Optimal Health Bullseye. The FHI is a compilation of health indicators that provide an insight into your current health status and potential for health concerns down the road. You will need a few minutes to sit down to complete the Index. I would encourage you to make a copy of this Index and give it to friends and family members. It is important to complete the Index before we move on because I find that most of us tend to think that we are healthier than we really are. Once we assign numbers, we put objectivity to the tool. The total number will show you how close you are to the Optimal Health Bullseye. Depending on your score, you will have to decide whether you want to improve or stay on a path toward illness and denial. If you have a higher score, your immune system is stressed and you will have a harder time facing the existing and new viruses, bacteria, and other pathogens, in addition to having a higher risk of chronic diseases.

When you go through the questions, don't spend too much time on any one question. If your answer is between two selections, skip it, fill out the other questions, and then go back. This will allow your brain time to process. Most likely, you will have a clear answer when you read that question again.

What is your Functional Health Index (FHI)?

Read the following statements and circle in the number that applies:
(How significant is the symptom? How true is the statement?)

KEY: 0 = No or Do not have the symptom, the symptom does not occur
1 = It is a minor or mild symptom, or it rarely occurs (once a month or less)
2 = It is a moderate symptom, or it occasionally occurs (weekly)
3 = It is a severe symptom, or it frequently occurs (daily)

Constipation or Diarrhea	0	1	2	3
Pass foul smelling gas	0	1	2	3
More than 3 or less than 1 bowel movements per day	0	1	2	3
Need to use antacids	0	1	2	3
Stomach bloating or feel sick after meals	0	1	2	3
Food sensitivities	0	1	2	3
Offensive breath	0	1	2	3
Heart palpitations	0	1	2	3
Heartburn	0	1	2	3
General Fatigue	0	1	2	3
Eating relieves fatigue	0	1	2	3
Decreased physical stamina	0	1	2	3
Hungry shortly after eating	0	1	2	3
Difficulty losing weight	0	1	2	3
Brain fog/difficult focusing	0	1	2	3
Getting up to urinate at night	0	1	2	3
Sleep less than 6 hours per night	0	1	2	3
Wake often during the night	0	1	2	3
Feel like you need to sleep more than 10 hours per night	0	1	2	3
Wake up in the morning unrested	0	1	2	1
Feel depressed	0	1	2	3
Take anti-depressants	0	1	2	3
Take prescription sleeping pills	0	1	2	3
Low sex drive	0	1	2	3

Female: periods lasting more than 5 days or abnormal cycle	0	1	2	3
Hot flashes	0	1	2	3
Facial hair growth	0	1	2	3
Unable to conceive	0	1	2	3
Male: Erectile dysfunction	0	1	2	3
Increased fat around the chest and hips	0	1	2	3
Hair loss	0	1	2	3
Athletes foot/Candida	0	1	2	3
Skin outbreaks, acne, rashes, dry skin, eczema, psoriasis or other fungus/yeast	0	1	2	3
Muscle cramping/twitching, day or night	0	1	2	3
Crave sweets or chocolate	0	1	2	3
Ache and pain throughout your body	0	1	2	3
Intolerance or loss of smells	0	1	2	3
Dizziness when standing up quickly	0	1	2	3
Swelling (edema) in ankles and wrists	0	1	2	3
Feel cold - hands and feet, all over	0	1	2	3
Thinning outer 1/3 of eyebrow	0	1	2	3
General headaches	0	1	2	3
Migraine headaches	0	1	2	3
Headache when waking in the morning or after a nap	0	1	2	3
Declining memory	0	1	2	3
High stress level	0	1	2	3
Feeling that life is unfulfilling	0	1	2	3
Difficulty calculating numbers	0	1	2	3
Multiple chemical sensitivities	0	1	2	3

Your Results
Total FHI = _____

0-5 POINTS

Congratulations are in order if you scored five or less. This is like throwing the ax and hitting the bullseye. I have found that the majority of patients with scores 5 and below are making good daily choices including healthy foods, regular exercise, supplements when needed, and carry low stress or have learned to modify their stress response in a positive manner. The focus of this group needs to be on prevention. For this group, I recommend yearly comprehensive blood work and the organic acids test. I also recommend for this group to have the genetic test. It is the most advanced test for staying healthy.

6-20 POINTS

If you scored between 6 and 20, you are better off than the average person. However, some modification is in order. In this second ring of the health bullseye, most people do not see their health as declining. You can still do pretty much everything you want to do with no restrictions. People in this group seem to catch a cold and whatever is going around more frequently. You might see less consistency in regular bowel movements. A lot of the symptoms are non-specific, but when you start putting them together, they become quite important. Persons scoring more towards 10 want to be aware that the slide to 20 can happen rather quickly, and with little warning. Oftentimes, this group has a diet that includes some fast food, sweets, and alcohol. Typically, the stress level is carried home from work or school and relationships can be tense at times, but you think that nothing needs to be done. Compared to your neighbors or fellow workers, you think you are pretty healthy. For this group, usually, biannual blood work and the organic acids test is the minimum to track specific progress and/or decline. Functional testing is the most important for this group because it identifies the underlying problems even when the patient cannot feel it. Changes toward optimal health occur more quickly compared to persons in the next two categories.

21-30 POINTS

Scores of 21 to 30 indicate that you need to get serious about finding out why your health is in this declining status and what changes need to be made to improve the course of your health. Many people in this category are starting to have a domino effect because of one condition causing or aggravating another condition. This group knows that they are not where they want to be but do not know what to do. They have been to doctors, they have tried a multitude of treatment options, and they are still running into the same problems. Frustration is a significant characteristic of people struggling in this category. If you are in this group, you know it is hard to make the best choices because you have tried so many things and nothing seems to work. I hear it often from patients and I understand that it is hard to think that another plan will make any difference. Don't give up! With the right tests and personal precision treatment, you can have your life back.

OVER 35 POINTS

If you have a score of more than 35, you need to call our office (406-998-1433) and set up an appointment ASAP for immediate consultation and testing. This is like throwing the ax and having it bounce off the wood backboard and land on the ground or throwing the ax and not even hitting the target. You have a major health crisis that can easily cause permanency if not reversed. Some people in this stage have already hit the point that significant turn-around is not possible. For those, the key is to prevent the condition from getting worse. This group of patients requires broad-based testing, both conventional and functional if they expect to reclaim their health. It can take several years of focused treatment to obtain optimal health, but improvements are often seen in as little as four to six weeks. I am sad to say that often people in this group do not believe they can get well and opt to stay in the dysfunctional health pattern. However, those who value their health wisely choose to go through the testing, focus on what they need to do, and then see their health and life restored. Below is a testimonial from someone who chose wisely:

TESTIMONIAL: KRIS

I am pleased to take this opportunity to express my appreciation to you for truly helping me, guiding me down a path to better health! I was really beginning to wonder if the age of 50 was the top of my mountain; that it was going to be all downhill from there. Thanks to you, I know that it is not the case at all! With your help, I truly feel like a new person; both physically and spiritually. It has been such a wonderful positive experience and such a blessing to know that there are doctors out there who genuinely care about their patients and desire for them to feel better.

I developed the FHI because there are significant numbers of people that either think or have been told that their symptoms are not important. They are often prescribed a drug to cover the symptoms, only to find out later that those symptoms were important. Chronic disease is rampant in this country; almost 50% of the adult population now has high blood pressure. Put a reminder in your calendar to score yourself every six months. If you would like our office to send you a reminder, go to www.goodmedicinefh.com and click on the "remind me" tab at the bottom of the page. The goal is to have the lowest score possible. It is a good way to track your overall health and know when to address issues as they arise to achieve the best consistent overall health. You have the power within you to start the change today.

Key Takeaways

- Symptoms alone are a poor way of assessing my health.

- My health is my choice.

- No matter where I score on the FHI, I can make improvements

- If I scored over 35 points, a full turn around may not be possible, but there is hope for improvement.

DR. GARY PETRO

Chapter Three

Test...Don't Guess

In this chapter, we will delve into the Optimal Health Analysis (OHA) method for determining the root cause of health conditions systematically and thoroughly. Over my many years of evaluating patients, I have used a lot of diagnostic tests and have watched the evolution of clinical testing. There are amazing tests available today; however, most doctors are not aware of them. Those that do stay up to date do not use them because often the insurance companies do not cover the advanced functional testing. You have to remember, your insurance company does not care if you live in optimal health; they are simply there to cover expenses per the policy limits. Essentially, they care about keeping you alive without regard to the quality of life you have. The human body is complex beyond comprehension. Think of your health as a puzzle; this new generation of appropriate and accurate testing helps fill in pieces of that puzzle. With the level of testing available today, guessing is not an option. Unfortunately, many chronic health conditions are still treated based on guesswork and intuition or with outdated testing.

There are a few assumptions that I am taking regarding this book:

- First, you do not have an immediately life-threatening disease.

- You have been to another doctor and had some tests run, usually a blood test.

- You have tried several treatment options on your own or at your physician's recommendation but keep returning out of frustration.

If all three of these assumptions are true, I can help you.

When you know your body is not functioning properly, but you don't know what to do, this disappointment can become overwhelming. It can lead to its own emotional and physical problems. Uncovering the underlying problems can be a difficult mission. However, the good news is that there are standard, functional, and genetic tests that can significantly help indicate what is wrong. Lab tests are continually being improved and new tests are being developed regularly. Most medical doctors lean heavily on blood tests. They can give excellent information—for some conditions, they can help rule out diagnoses—but often they do little to determine what is causing a patient's problem.

Most of the patients I see have had only minimal blood panels run over and over. Having seen thousands and thousands of patients, I can say that most of them had several abnormal lab findings that were not considered significant by the ordering doctor. The patient was never even notified of the results or was told not to worry about them. This sheds light on the current state of our health care system. If you have abnormal findings, unless your physician takes a functional system approach, there is little that can be done other than wait for it to get worse or cover the symptom with drugs. The condition continues to worsen, bringing with it more health issues, and frequently, a shortened lifespan. The Functional Medicine approach is to identify dysfunctional body systems and treat at the lowest level to prevent further health decline and to up-regulate the body's defense systems.

HOMEOSTASIS

To understand how Functional Medicine identifies these dysfunctional body systems, we first need to understand these systems. The automatic control of our body's systems is called homeostasis. The Biology Dictionary defines homeostasis as:

"the balance within a system that keeps it operating within a range of conditions. Homeostasis helps us maintain stable internal and external environments with the best conditions for it to operate. It is a dynamic process that requires constant monitoring of all systems in the body to detect changes, and mechanisms that react to those changes and restore stability".[9]

Homeostasis is kind of like the heating system in your house or apartment. Let's say you want it to be 75 degrees, so you turn the thermostat to 75 degrees. If the room is 65 degrees, the thermostat triggers the furnace to start generating heat until the temperature reaches 75 degrees. Then the thermostat turns off the furnace. When the temperature in the room dips a few degrees, the furnace will turn on again to keep the temperature right around 75 degrees.

Similarly, our body uses a regulating system for every part of our body. When these regulating systems fail to function optimally, health issues start to develop. These systems are highly developed and controlled by your brain and neuroendocrine pathways, from your genetic blueprint.

Now, let's look at what happens in the stomach when this automatic system does not work correctly. It is estimated that 10-20% of the western world is affected by GERD (Gastric Esophageal Reflux Disease) and 40% have heartburn one or more times a week. The regulation system of the stomach is intended to keep an acidity of about 1.8 pH. If we take antacids or proton pump inhibitors (Zantac, Nexium, Prevacid, etc.), this system is now altered, and the thermostat-like control is not going to work properly. This is like turning the thermostat up to 75 degrees and the furnace kicks on, however, when the temperature in the room reaches 75, the furnace keeps on forcing out the heat. Now you need to open the windows and door or turn the furnace off manually. The drugs mentioned above were designed to be taken for 12 weeks or less. In my practice, most people I see who are on these drugs have been on them for many years. Taking them for a short period will most likely cause minimal problems, but many patients take them on an ongoing basis.

This is an example of the symptoms being controlled with drugs instead of balancing the system. The decreased acid can cause a host of potential problems including stomach cancers, bone fractures, impaired absorption of micronutrients, kidney disease, increased risk of infections, and is now even linked to cardiovascular death.[10]

Another example of homeostasis in action is that, when we eat, if there is not enough acid to break down the food as it is combined with enzymes and digestive secretions, a signal will be sent to produce more digestive secretions. The parietal and chief cells in the lining of the stomach will then start producing more hydrochloric acid and enzymes to digest the food before it moves into the small intestine. This is a great system and should work similarly to a thermostat. It is all under neurological and genetic control. If there is not enough acid in the stomach as the food enters, a signal causes more acid to be produced and often produces excess acid, like the furnace not shutting off. The additional acid can enter the lower part of the esophagus and cause erosion, scarring, and heartburn. This often leads the lower esophagus to become narrowed from the scarring and leads to difficulty swallowing.

The functional approach to this is to ask a series of questions. Are there any foreign bacteria, yeast, virus, or parasites causing abnormal digestive function? Is the patient under abnormal stress? What are their dietary habits, including caffeine? Depending on age, is there a genetic concern for possible future stomach cancer? Then we can start with simple protocols:

- Gargling with water for one minute twice a day to stimulate the vagus nerve that affects the function of the stomach

- Specific exercises including strength and modified aerobic

- Stress reduction techniques

- Drinking lemon water, apple cider vinegar, or taking a weak gastric acid supplement just before a meal to mildly increase the acid but not enough to cause an overproduction of acid

- After a few weeks, we may discuss the addition of digestive enzymes, probiotics, magnesium, if the test indicates the need

As you can see, this approach works with your body to cause adjustment of the regulation mechanism with the goal of eventual control through a diet and other lifestyle activities.

Most of the people who I consult with have had little testing or the wrong kind of testing. Most have been put on generalized treatment plans that help some but fall short of helping most. Since we are all genetically different, doesn't it make sense that each of us might require different treatment plans?

OUR HEALTH AS AN APPLE TREE

Let's use an apple tree as an analogy representing our health. We are hungry and eating an apple sounds good. So, we go out looking for an apple tree. We see one in the distance that looks strong, with no large broken branches, the leaves look green, and we can see a good number of red apples weighing down the branches. As we get close to the tree, it doesn't look quite as good. Some of the bark is missing around the trunk, the leaves that looked so green from a distance have yellow and some brown around the edges and their backsides have yellowish-green bumps. The apples are red but are not uniform and do not have the vibrant red that is typical of this variety of apples. We pick one and take a bite. We are surprised that it does not have the crisp texture that we expected at harvest time. Most people would prefer not to eat apples from this tree because they are not of the high quality one would expect. The apples are not rotten, worm-eaten, nor do they have a blight. These apples would most likely be sold by the orchard to local stores, or a wholesaler because they look acceptable enough on the outside. However, we would not pick this apple when a much more delicious one is in the same bin. This apple is considered sub-optimal but good enough to be sold.

For many people around the world—and especially in the U.S.—this is their health status: sub-optimal, able to get through, but lacking the appeal of the shiny, delicious, crunchy apple we desire. I believe, if most of us are honest, we want exceptionally good health.

So, we need to ask a few questions. Why didn't this apple develop properly? Could it be the cold spring temperatures, or the drought that happened mid-summer, and then excessive rain after? Could it be the aerial spraying of other crops in the area on a windy day? Or a depletion of required nutrients from improper crop rotation of neighboring fields? The questions could go on and on, but without proper testing, we would never know why. Luckily, for the human body, we have functional health tests that can give an insight into the "what" and "why" of dysfunctional health.

TESTS AND THEIR MEANING

In my clinical opinion, the tests make the difference between treating a condition and treating a person. Because of our genetic distinctiveness, the specific tests show how that individuality expresses how one feels daily. Reading through lab manuals can be quite tedious for many people, however, I find them quite interesting. Many of my lab manuals and reference texts are well worn! Instead of boring you with the specific numbers though, I am just going to go through several of the most important blood tests and explain their significance. If this is more information that you want at this point, feel free to just skip to the next section.

My process of ordering tests is to keep the information stream as specific to a patient as possible. There is no reason to run a large battery of tests when I know that, for most patients, most of the information will be negative. This is what confuses me when looking at patients with health problems that have had the same test run every six months, only to get the same results.

Most everyone reading this book has had at least one blood draw in their life. More likely, you have had many blood draws over the years. Blood work is a double-edged sword. Its interpretation can either be a great aid to solving a person's health problems or it can give a false sense of well-being. If you are like many patients, you have your blood taken regularly—yearly, every six months, or every month, depending on whether you have any symptoms or not. I often review the last few years of a patient's labs before their consultation. I have the unfortunate obligation to tell many patients that things do not look as good as they have been told.

You might wonder why this is the case. There are two reasons:

1. Blood work, like all testing, is like putting a puzzle together. Some tests by themselves give significant detail. Yet other tests need to be viewed as part of a process or algorithm and alone will not indicate a specific condition.

2. Standard normal lab values do not represent functional values. A normal value at one lab can be abnormal at another. Abnormal lab values are determined mathematically at labs by taking all the samples of a specific test in a given time period and calculating the upper and lower 2.5%. The highest 2.5% is deemed to be abnormally high lab values and the lowest 2.5% is the range for abnormally low values. Some of the standard lab values will be similar to the optimal levels, but others have deviated because the general population's health has declined, and the calculations have deviated with the declining health. If you read the information of most labs, they will express that a normal test does not promise good health and that an abnormal result does not mean you are sick. Reference ranges are based on statistics of a group of presumed healthy individuals.

So, tests can be a little more complicated than we are sometimes led to believe. As a patient, you do not need to understand every specific test. However, it is important to realize that there are specific lab tests that are beneficial to finding the underlying problems for your health.

BLOOD TESTS RESULTS

This is not a lab manual, so I will keep the points brief. I have included optimal values if you want to compare your prior tests. Blood tests are by far the most used of any diagnostic procedure. More physicians are becoming aware of the possibility of false-positive results from blood work. Many times, blood tests are being run routinely to find something abnormal, rather than being run to confirm a condition.[11] As part of the OHA (Optimal Health Analysis), blood work is an important way to look for alarms and missed indicators. The following are some of my routine blood tests that give the most information.

Test	Optimal Level	Normal Lab level	Comments/Symptoms
Glucose	75-90 mg/dL	65-99 mg/dL	Primary sugar that fuels our brain and body. Symptoms of low glucose: fatigue, anxiety, irritability, mental confusion, and blurred vision. Symptoms of elevated glucose include fatigue, headaches, blurred vision, frequent urination, increased thirst, abdominal pain, confusion, difficulty concentrating. Glucose levels are affected by carbohydrate intake, stress, hormone, and
Pre-diabetes	100-125 mg/dL		
Diabetes	126+ mg/dL		

			liver function.
Hemoglobin A1C	<5.2%	<5.7%	Indicator of blood sugar over the past 3-4 months. It is also used to indicate treatment effectiveness.
Pre-diabetes	5.7-6.4%	>5.7-6.4%	
Diabetes	>6.5%	>6.5%	
Inflammation Markers			
CRP-hs	0-.5 mg/dL	0-.8 mg/dl	C Reactive Protein (high sensitivity) is one of the best measures for inflammation. It is made in the liver and elevates during inflammation conditions, as in acute trauma, infection, autoimmune conditions, food allergy, or sensitivities. It indicates inflammation but not where.
Homocysteine	0-6 umol/L	0-10.3 umol/L	Higher levels increase the risk for cardiovascular disease
ESR	0-10mm/hr	0-20 mm/hr	Non-specific marker for inflammation.
Magnesium	2.2-2.6 mg/dL	1.6-2.6 mg/dL	It is responsible for being part of over 350 biochemical reactions in the human body. Standard magnesium levels often do not give an accurate indication of magnesium levels, a more advanced and accurate test is an intracellular magnesium blood test. Your

			morning urine pH test is also a good indicator of magnesium levels. Deficiency symptoms include heart arrhythmia (uneven heart rate), decreased appetite, mental confusion, loose bowel, fatigue, muscle cramps, and irritability.
Liver Tests			
AST (SGOT)	10-26 IU/L	10-35 IU/L	Primarily used to determine liver stress/damage. The organic acid test is more specific for functional testing, except for extremely high blood levels that need to be referred for medical evaluation and crisis treatment. Symptoms relating to liver disease abnormalities can include fatigue/weakness, jaundice, abdominal pain/swelling, nausea, vomiting, itching, light-colored bowel movement, loss of appetite.
ALT (SGPT)	10-26 IU/L	6-29 IU/L	
GGT	10-30 IU/L	3-70 IU/L	Most is concentrated in the liver but also in the pancreas, spleen, and kidney. ALT alone will be elevated in bone disease, however, GGT and ALT will both be elevated in liver disease. Other than that, it is not a useful test. It can

			also indicate a reduction in glutathione levels; however, organic acid tests will usually give more accurate information regarding glutathione dysfunction.
Calcium	9.4-10.1 mg/dL	8.7-10.2 mg/dL	Important for the nerve function, heart, muscles, bone formation, and blood clotting. Only about 50% of the calcium ingested is absorbed. That which is absorbed needs vitamin D and is under the regulation of the parathyroid hormone. Blood pH levels can also affect calcium levels.
Iron Tests	Four tests make up a standard iron panel. Through an evaluation matrix, the tests can indicate several issues that can contribute to many of the symptoms commonly expressed by patients today.		Symptoms of iron deficiency can include fatigue, headaches weakness, chest pain, burning tongue, dizziness, fingernail spooning, leg pain, memory deficit, shortness of breath, cravings for dirt or chalk. Symptoms of iron overload (excess iron) can cause fatigue, memory deficit, low sex drive, weakness, joint pain, jaundice, symptoms of heart disease.
TIBC (Total Binding Iron Capacity)	250-350 ug/d	250-425 ug/d	The amount of iron bound to protein in the blood.

Serum Iron	85-130 ug/dL	40-160 ug/dL	Indicates transition time between iron depletion and the development of anemia. Increased levels associated with liver dysfunction.
Ferritin	40-150 ug/dL	10-232 ug/dL	Ferritin is the most accurate marker of the amount of iron stored in your body.
Iron Saturation	24-50%	15-50%	Sensitive test for iron deficiency.
Electrolytes			
Sodium	135-142 mEq/L	135-146 MEq/L	Electrolytes form a delicate balance within the body. Imbalance can be indicators of many disease processes too numerous to detail here.
Potassium	4.0-4.5 mEq/L	3.5-5.3 mEq/L	
Chloride	100-106 mEq/L	98-110 mEq/L	
CO2	25-30 mWq/L	19-30 mEq/L	
Thyroid			All the thyroid tests are important, but the following are the key tests:
TSH	1.0-3.0 uU/mL	.45-5.5 uU/mL	Thyroid-stimulating hormone is released from your pituitary gland to communicate with your thyroid.
Reverse T3	9.2-24.1 ng/DL	8-25 ng/DL	Chronic stress and high cortisol can raise levels of reverse T3, which is an unusable form of the thyroid hormone. RT3 is like the brake of the thyroid.
Thyroid Peroxidase	<9 IU/ml	<9 IU/ml	High levels of thyroid antibodies show an

(TPO)			autoimmune attack against the
Thyroglobulin Ab	<4 IU/ml	<4 IU/ml	thyroid. The overwhelming majority of positive thyroid cases are on the autoimmune spectrum, the most common being Hashimoto's disease.
Lipid Panel			
Total Cholesterol	155-200 mg/dL	125-200 mg/dL	The backbone of all steroid hormones in the body. The liver, skin, and intestines produce 60-80% of the body's cholesterol, 20-40% from diet. Often associated with thyroid conditions, liver disease, gall bladder problems, and heavy metals. Can contribute to cardiovascular disease.
HDL	55-70 mg/dL	46-100 mg/dL	"Good cholesterol" Transports cholesterol to the liver for processing.
Triglycerides	50-100 mg/dL	0-150 mg/dL	Often increase with cardiovascular disease, hypothyroidism, adrenal dysfunction, metabolic syndrome, and others.
Protein level	6.9-7.4 g/dL	6.10-8.10 g/dL	Total protein, which is comprised of roughly 60% Albumin and 40% Globulin. Protein is necessary for making muscle tissue and they are broken down to amino acids as they flow through the stomach and small intestine. Hydrochloric acid is secreted

				in the stomach as well as pancreatic enzymes in the small intestine. Symptoms relating to protein abnormalities can include fatigue, weight fluctuations, edema, muscle weakness, and loss.

*   Most standard lipid panels only include a mathematical calculated LDL and not an actual LDL level.
*   Certain test results are gender-specific; listed values are general in nature.

ORGANIC ACID TESTING

The next component of the OHA is organic acid testing. Organic acids are chemical compounds excreted in the urine that provide unique insights into the body's cellular metabolic processes. In the U.S., organic acid tests are performed on almost every newborn before leaving the hospital to screen for specific diseases. Organic acids are derived from the metabolic conversion of proteins, fats, and carbohydrates, in addition to compounds of bacterial origin. The test is performed from a simple urine sample because the concentrations are 100 times that of a blood sample. Since the use of the test began, researchers have found over 1,000 different organic acids. This is, by far, the most important of the initial tests that I order for my patients. The organic acid test gives detailed information about cellular energy production, carbohydrate metabolism, fat metabolism, methylation, detoxification, brain chemistry, digestive dysfunction, oxidation, and amino acid regulation. With the organic acids test, I can drill down quickly to see what organ systems are involved to streamline follow-up testing.

CASE STUDY: AMBER

Amber came in as a patient complaining of significant fatigue for the past several years. She was a young mother of three. She was frustrated because she tried to eat well, get enough sleep at night, and go to the gym at least three times a week. She said her marriage was good and she experienced the usual stress at work. The harder she tried, the more fatigued she became. She had been to several other physicians and felt herself barely keeping up with her life's demands. I reviewed her blood work from the previous year, and nothing stood out. I explained that there was a good chance that her mitochondria—a part of the nucleus of each cell that makes energy for the body—were not functioning properly. We ran the organic acid test. The results indicated that not only were the mitochondria underperforming but she also did not have enough mitochondria. We put her on a treatment protocol including free form amino acids, CoQ10, magnesium, Vitamin C, and two specialized mitochondrial supplements. She was also instructed to back off on her exercise routines to keep her heart rate at no more than 70% of her maximum. Within 2-3 weeks, Amber started feeling like she had some margin in her life. At the two-month point, she said her energy was back to 80% of normal, at which time I increased her exercise to include resistive training as well as aerobic activity. At her next follow-up appointment, she felt like she was back to her old self and was released to return to full exercise.

STOOL TESTING

The next test in the OHA is a DNA/PCR stool sample (poop test). Colonoscopies are done frequently within conventional medicine. They can be good for identifying late stages of disease, nodules, and anatomical issues but do not address the metabolism and underlying early- and mid-stage gut issues. Stool testing is not a topic that most people like to think about, however, the specialized stool tests that I use give information about what is and what is not working in your gut. The digestive system (also called your gut) is considered the second brain of the body and the most overworked organ system. The nerves called the enteric nervous system—located in the abdominal area—have about the same number of nerve cells as the spinal cord and your gut has an immense impact on your health. It affects your brain chemistry and immune system and is intertwined with every other system that makes you function. The number of patients that come in with GI problems keeps climbing due to our lifestyles and our genetic variations. Currently, over 60% of the U.S. population has digestive issues. The advanced stool testing I use allows me to assess digestive and absorptive functions, detect pathogens and parasites, and identify specific bacteria and yeasts. The biggest problem with conventional stool testing is some of the organisms keep growing and others die in the transit time between when the sample is taken and when the hospital or lab receives it.

This can cause errors resulting in inappropriate treatment based on poor data. The primary stool test I use is extremely sensitive. It uses a technology called MALDI-TOF MS (Matrix-Assisted Laser Desorption Ionization-Time of Flight Mass Spectrometry). It is FDA approved and will be used in all hospitals and clinical labs in the future.

The organisms die immediately when the sample is placed in a collection solution. When it arrives at the lab, the molecular fingerprint of the 7,000+ organisms is compared to the sample and reported. Once we know what is or is not there, the 4 R's (Remove, Replace, Re-Inoculate, and Repair) can be targeted. I find that gut symptoms often start changing within a few weeks after treatment begins. And that is a welcome change for my patients.

CASE STUDY: SAM

Sam's mother brought him into the office. He was an energetic 14-year-old boy. His mother went on to tell me that he was having such foul-smelling bowel gas on the school bus on the way home from school that the other students were complaining. This had gone on for several months, and now even the bus driver was taking issue. They had already been to their medical doctor and tried a few treatments without success. I studied his diet, which was rather good, and decided to run a detailed stool test. The results came back showing an imbalance of good bacteria and some opportunistic bacteria. I placed him on a special probiotic to increase the good bacteria in the lower colon without affecting the bacteria in the small intestine. At his follow-up appointment a month later, his mother said the bus driver and fellow students were grateful.

GENETIC TESTING

The OHA would not be possible without genetic testing. Genetic testing is the exciting future of health care. With one cheek swab, I can see your genetic footprint and almost every known mutation that has been scientifically shown to have an impact on your current and future health, as well as the degree of impact of that variation. Our genes do not change throughout life, so all that is needed is one sample. Did you know that we all have 99.9% of the same genes? The variation, or mutation, of the genes is what makes us look, act, and function differently. Most of the time, I do not focus on specific genes but rather on families and groups of genes with sophisticated AI (artificial intelligence) software called Opus23. It is a suite of applications that allows me to import raw genomic data and perform a series of extraordinarily sophisticated analytics on it.

This testing has made it possible to look at each patient's individual differences and apply treatment based on your own genes, for specificity that was not possible before. I use this testing for two different purposes:

1. The first application is for people who struggle with their health and have tried several treatments without resolution. The results are usually eye-opening to the patient and allow me to give personalized, precision recommendations.

2. The other category is for extremely healthy persons who want to stay healthy. I can get information from their genetic blueprint that can help prevent disease that is coded in their genes. Many of the degenerative diseases take years to develop before any symptoms appear. When we can identify these gene alterations and make preventative changes through lifestyle, the patient has the greatest opportunity to avoid these diseases and to live life optimally. With this test, I can identify patients who are prone to physical as well as emotional problems. For example, if you have a family history of Alzheimer's or other neurodegenerative diseases, you need to be checked for the likelihood of developing those diseases later in life. Imagine what can happen when we work at truly preventing disease instead of just treating it!

CASE STUDY: LISA

Lisa was a kind, middle-aged woman who came in for general fatigue, chest pain, high cholesterol, and digestive issues. She worked at a medical facility but also had been involved with natural treatment for many years including essential oils and nutritional supplementation. She was very frustrated because she knew she should be feeling better. She had recently been in the hospital for evaluation of her heart, but they were not able to find any reason for her symptoms other than possibly the elevated cholesterol. Her symptoms had been progressing for several years and she wanted change. Her history revealed she had been under significant stress with family issues for many years. I decided to run the genetics test because she was doing so much right already. In four weeks, the data came back, and I started putting it through the Opus 23 evaluation platforms. A significant number of abnormal SNPs* showed a high probability of altered genetic function. She had several cardiac gene SNPs indicating she had a 635% increased chance of Coronary Artery Disease (CAD), and increased risk of an aneurism. It also showed that her mitochondria, which produce energy in the cells, had mutations not allowing B6 to be synthesized properly. Additionally, she had a gene variation that was not allowing the proper processing of folic acid. This was interesting because the more common MTHFR gene was working fine. Changes were made to her diet along with supplementation and stress control activities. Within six weeks, she was gaining her lost energy. She was still not able to do resistance exercise but was walking five days a week. She had not reported any recurrent chest pain and her digestive issues were minimal.

*A single nucleotide polymorphism (SNPs) is the most common genetic variation. They can affect the gene's function causing altered cell activity.

I, like most functional physicians, have many additional tests at my disposal depending on a patient's complaints, age, and other known health conditions. I have found that the OHA gives the greatest amount of clinical information with the fewest tests.

Functional testing is the key to linking your symptoms to effective, precise treatment. Without functional tests, the only way to treat is with general protocols that can be effective for some but are nonspecific, and without precision.

Key Takeaways

- The OHA (Optimal Health Analysis) method of testing is essential for a thorough health evaluation.

- If my blood work keeps coming back normal and I am having symptoms, I need to have functional testing.

- Appropriate testing is an effective way to understand underlying health problems.

- The organic acid test is a simple urine test that scans a wide range of cellular conditions.

- My gut is considered the second brain to my body, so stool testing can be immensely helpful.

- Genetic testing is essential for health conditions that are not responding to appropriate care.

Chapter Four

The World of Genomics and Precision Medicine

*Our genes load the gun,
our lifestyle pulls the trigger.*

There is no one else exactly like you. Individuality is who we are--our looks, emotions, what drives us, how we respond to certain foods, drugs, how we sleep, etc. If you are like most people, someone has come up to you at some point and said, "you look just like ___." That is because we all share 99.9% of the same genes. It is that .1% that gives us our uniqueness, our individuality. We now have cost-effective technology that allows anyone to have their genes tested. Genetic testing gives us accurate information that can help us live healthier, longer, and with greater enjoyment in life.

For example, Alzheimer's disease is growing at a fast pace. It is the fifth-leading cause of death among those age 65 and older and is also is a top cause of disability and poor health. The National Institute of Health now states that a combination of age-related changes in the brain—along with genetic, environmental, and lifestyle factors—is the most likely reason for the increase. Interesting! That sounds like what I have been saying about all health conditions! What people are not hearing, though, is the ability to abort, minimize, or delay the onset of Alzheimer's through proper testing and natural treatment. Take, for example, the Apolipoprotein E4 (APOE) gene, which is an extraordinarily strong risk factor for the disease. If you have one copy of that gene, you have a 30% risk; if you have two copies, that risk goes up to 60%. Now, research has shown that using precision medicine based on genomic data, we can impact the disease by applying proper nutrition, exercise, and emotional techniques to decrease brain inflammation. I believe most people would want to know this information and to be able to reduce the risks, keep their memory, and reduce the impact on their family both emotionally and financially. Before genomics, Alzheimer's disease was thought to be a result of genetic inheritance. Now we know better. If you have a family history of Alzheimer's, call or email us to schedule the appropriate testing.

When I look at a person's genetic data, I am looking at the gene variation called Single Nucleotide Polymorphism (SNP), pronounced "snip." Each SNP represents a difference in a single DNA building block, called a nucleotide.[12] I often get questions about the direct-to-consumer genetic testing that is available online.

It was difficult to watch TV in the past several years without seeing the ads for 23andMe and Ancestry.com. 23andMe alone has over 10 million customers! Remarkably, one of the co-founders was married to the founder of Google. The business model of 23andMe was to sell test kits below what it actually costs to process the genetic information and give a watered-down report to the consumer, all while amassing huge amounts of genetic data to partner with innovative research and development for novel medications. Due to FDA regulations, more detailed genetic information that could indicate significant diseases was not allowed to be reported to the consumer by companies like 23andMe. In 2018, GlaxoSmithKline invested 300 million dollars into 23andMe so they could use the genetic information of its 10 million consumers. Since then, 23andMe has significantly reduced the amount of genetic data that is analyzed, including many of the important SNPs.

The chip or sample source that I currently use in genetic testing includes over 900,000 SNPs, including most of the important SNPs that were deleted from the direct to consumer platforms. The AI programs that I use curate more than 6,000 genetic alterations that are useful today. Of the 2,500 that are of clinical interest, over 700 revolve around medication reaction, and an additional 3,000 have to do with potential diseases. This gives me a robust platform to help steer patients toward optimal health.

On October 1st, 2015, we celebrated an important milestone. It was the 25th anniversary of the Human Genome Project. You might ask why this is important. Well, the Human Genome Project is the genetic blueprint map for you and me and every other human being. Before the project, it was thought that humans had between 100,000-200,000 genes because of our extreme complexity. The research was conducted as a collaborative program with the goal of completely mapping and understanding all human genes. In the journal *Nature* in 2001, the initial draft of the human genome was published by the International Human Genome Sequencing Consortium. It was an estimated 90% complete. They were startled to find that the total number of genes was much lower than the original estimates, at around 30,000 genes. When the project was finished, it was concluded that there are only around 21,000 genes in a human being. Comparing between humans and mice, they found that we share about 97.5% of the same working DNA. According to scientists at both Stanford University of Medicine and Yale University, the interaction of the sequences with a class of proteins, called transcription factors, can be the reason we see the vast differences between people. This can account for our appearances, development, and predisposition to certain diseases. Therefore, identical twins can have different abilities, diseases, and—ultimately—looks, as they age. We have over 200 cell types in the body and, amazingly, each cell interprets this identical genetic information very differently to carry out the functions necessary to keep us alive.

Looking at a single gene variation provides little information except for certain genetic diseases that affect a minute percentage of the population. However, analyzing groups and families of genes can have a profound effect on helping patients find the missing links of health information for which they have been searching. The emerging area of genomic health is one of the most exciting for me.

Genetics often looks at specific genes having to do with congenital disorders like muscular dystrophy, cystic fibrosis, etc., whereas genomics is concerned with how your genes affect your body's response to food, medication, supplements, and the environment around you. For me, this genomic component has made a quantum shift in my ability to evaluate a patient's health problems. I can drill down to the specific details of a patient's uniqueness. Never before have we been able to cost-effectively look with detail at metabolic function on an individual basis.

So, when I consult a new patient that has tried a wide variety of treatment options without success, a genetic test is essential. I know some critical bits of information have been missed. Instead of re-doing the same battery of tests, I want to see what genetic variations they have that could be influencing their symptoms. This information, combined with the other functional testing, is a great one-two punch. The reality is, some of you were born with a better gene pool than others and require less modification for your body to adapt.

EPIGENETICS: WHY WE ARE THE WAY WE ARE

I started studying epigenetics roughly eight years ago and the intrigue propelled me to dig deeper into genetics. While genetics is the analysis of genes and inheritance, Epigenetics is the study of how environmental factors switch genes on and off. It determines which proteins are transcribed to make us who we are. The utterly amazing part is the sequencing that controls the DNA. It has been said that the genome is like the hardware of a computer and the epigenome is more related to the software that signals the computer when to work, how much, and what to focus on. Gene function can be altered by more than just changing sequence; the greater system relates to turning the genes on and off through methylation. The first human disease that was linked to epigenetics was cancer in 1983.

Let's look at the Agouti mouse for an example of epigenetics. The Agouti mouse is bred for research. All Agouti mice have identical DNA, so they all have the same genomes as each other. They have been bred to have an inherently high risk for cholesterol, diabetes, overweight, yellow fur, and high tumor risk.

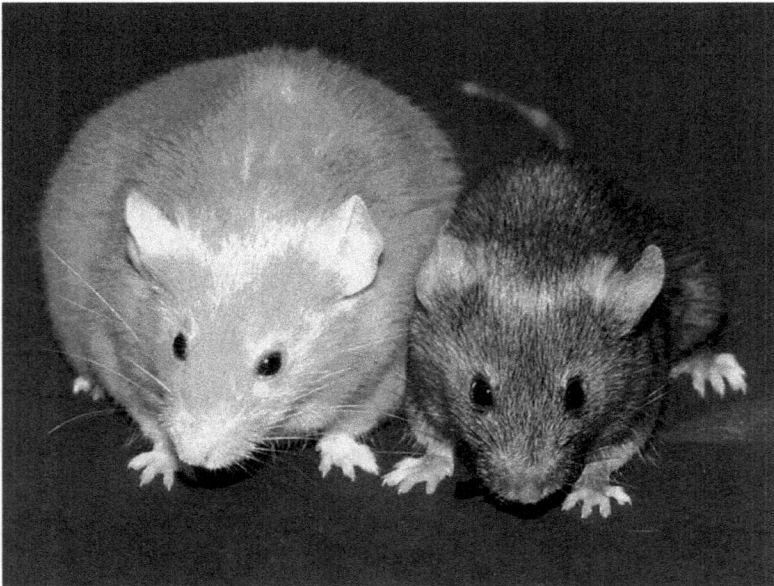

Agouti Mouse

Credit: © Dana Dolinoy, University of Michigan, Ann Arbor, and Randy Jirtle, Duke University, Durham, NC

In a reproducible experiment, a pregnant Agouti mouse is given daily supplements of Vitamin B12, folic acid, choline, and betaine (from sugar beets). The offspring grow to have primarily brown fur, are smaller, and have a decreased risk for diabetes, cancer, and elevated cholesterol. Another pregnant Agouti mouse is not given any supplements or altered lifestyle. Her offspring are born with primarily yellow fur and grow to have a higher risk of diabetes, cancer, and are overweight.

In another test, the researcher allowed a pregnant mouse to be exposed to bisphenol A (BPA), a synthetic compound in many plastic items including plastic drinking bottles. Most of the offspring were born with yellow fur, high tumor, and diabetes rates. So, how does this happen? Research shows that methylation is the reason for these changes.[13] (Methylation is a way of turning genes on and off. This process can change the activity of a portion of DNA without changing the sequence or structure.) There is now evidence that autoimmune diseases, congenital disorders, and certain cancers are caused, to a high degree, due to the lack of methylation. It has also been shown that these negative changes can carry through multiple generations. The exciting part is that nutritional supplementation can reverse the process. As in the case of the Agouti mice, when I evaluate the genome of patients, I often see significant issues regarding the methylation system map.

Epigenetics is considered to be the missing link between nature and nurture. There is a significant indication that the risk of many chronic adult diseases and health disorders results from exposure to environmental factors early in development. Just this week, a new research report was published showing that Celiac disease is attributable to environmental factors, specifically pesticides, and chemicals.[14] The report goes on to state that genetic modification is particularly susceptible to changes during pregnancy, neonatal development, puberty, and old age.

GENES, CONCEPTION, AND HEALTH

It is always important to be optimally healthy, but the most important time is before conception. Healthy parents will give the baby the best opportunity for the best gene pool possible. The better the genes, the less risk of disease, both at birth and later in life.[15] All humans have 23 chromosomes. The sex of a baby is determined by the X and Y chromosomes. An XY set develops as a male and an XX as a female. Half of your chromosomes come from your mother and half from your father or sperm donor. Other species have different numbers of chromosomes. For example, a dog has 39 pairs, a mosquito has 3 pairs, and a rice plant has 12 pairs. Within the roughly 25,000 human genes are 3 million base pairs. Some of the genes are made of only a few hundred base pairs and others more than 2 million pairs. The point is it is a complex system and multiple small changes can significantly impact our health and longevity. People that have a more robust gene pool can have fewer health issues, and generally, a longer life. Studies of people in their 90s, 100s, 105-109s, and those over 110, show that this extended life span has little to do with income, education, or profession. It has much to do with lifestyle. These people consistently were nonsmokers, cope well with stress, are not obese, and are active for their age. Most of these people are women and are less prone to develop age-related chronic diseases like high blood pressure, cancer, diabetes, and heart disease because of their lifestyle choices.

Each generation is born with both new and inherited gene mutations. You have a different combination than your parents and your children have a different set of genetic variations than you. Some are harmless and others can end life early. The probability is even worse when the mother has a poor lifestyle during the time from conception to early pregnancy. This critical period can substantially alter an offspring's chance for an optimal life. If you are thinking about having a child, some of my best advice is to get as healthy as you can. I do not just mean looking good but having your body function optimally. Your baby will appreciate it later in life. The OHA process is excellent to determine where improvement needs to be focused.

In the US, more parents are now having babies in their 30s than in their 20s, according to the Centers for Disease Control (CDC). Birth defects, as well as mutations in the DNA, increase as the parents' age increases. Women are aware of the changes in their bodies that make getting pregnant more difficult after approximately age 35. However, there is a greater chance for babies conceived by fathers over the age of 45 to experience premature birth, late stillbirth, decreased Apgar scores, low birth weight, newborn seizures, and birth defects such as congenital heart defects and cleft palate. As these infants grow into childhood, they have an increased chance of childhood cancers, autisms, as well as schizophrenia, and cognitive disorders. These are results of genetic damage of which parents need to be aware. Fertility traits in humans are also under genetic control. It can be devastating for a couple when they are not able to have a child, but instead of asking why the couple is having a problem conceiving, the standard approach is to look at In vitro fertilization (IVF). Besides being very costly, IVF increases the offspring's risk later in life of having hypertension, vascular dysfunction, diabetes, and obesity.

CASE STUDY: REBECCA AND JACOB

Rebecca was a kind, petite Amish woman in her early 20s married to a man named Jacob. Rebecca had had three miscarriages in the prior two years and was given no hope. Having children, raising them, and socialization with neighbors and relatives are the greatest functions of the Amish family, so not having children was putting huge stress on the couple. After assessing Rebecca's hormone, stress, and nutritional levels, I placed her on a specific treatment protocol to up-regulate the depressed hormones and balance her liver and neurotransmitters. Within six months, she conceived, and she and Jacob had a healthy baby boy. They went on to have two additional children in the next few years. Rebecca and Jacob felt like they truly were part of their community again.

Almost 20% of all pregnancies now end in miscarriage.[16] Using the OHA method for testing, combined with a functional model to treat women with difficulty conceiving, can be highly effective. Most of the time, it is not difficult to identify the system or systems that are affecting the hormone balance. I treat to up- or down-regulate the poorly working systems and then allow the body to function as designed.

ONE SIZE DOES NOT FIT ALL

You might have heard of Curcumin, which is the active ingredient in turmeric, a powerful supplement. It is one of the most researched nutritional agents. Curcumin reduces inflammation, works as an antioxidant, and decreases cancer, to name a few of the amazing qualities of curcumin. For many people, it can be extremely beneficial. However, for others, it can cause negative effects on their health. That is how genetics works. Our genes determine how we respond to everything. I have known this intuitively, but now we have the tools to put this concept into practice. It is one of the main reasons why one size does not fit all. It makes no difference if we are talking about medication, nutritional supplementation, exercise, sleep protocol, or stress-relieving tools. What works very well for your friend at work or neighbor can have an adverse effect on you.

In summary, let's imagine we are going to the planetarium. You find yourself getting comfortable in the reclining chair. As the show starts, the lights dim. The sun is setting in the west and we see the moon increasing in intensity. The sky transitions to a medium blue and we can start to see a few planets and stars appear. Soon, we see multiple planets and stars emerge as the sun has fully set. It's an amazing sight. Think about this as representing the tools physicians have had to diagnose patients. Included are blood work, CT & MRI scans, functional tests, biopsies, and physical tests, to name a few. The excitement starts here: as the lights dim to total darkness, the heavenly realm is visible. The vast array of planets, stars, and galaxies appear. The presenter points his light pen to take our attention to different star formations, and then to the immense galaxies. We are blown away by the vastness and how they are all in relative position to one another as we think of the width and breadth of the universe. This point in the planetarium show represents this new arena of genomics. There are millions of possibilities that are set in place by your genetic blueprint. This new testing is blowing open the ability to give patients personalized, precision treatment rather than simply using standardized treatment plans.

I have been told by pharmaceutical developers that, eventually, medication will be much more targeted, based on a patient's genetic results. This will be a big win for patients, meaning fewer side effects, a greater chance of effectiveness, and minimal tragic losses.[17] With our individual uniqueness properly understood, we can all be treated differently, just as we should be.

Key Takeaways:

- Genetic testing can be a gamechanger.

- My genes do not change throughout my life.

- I can—directly and indirectly—affect the expression of my genes throughout lifestyle habits.

- Genetic testing provides necessary information for precision personalized treatment.

- Genetic SNPs have a significant impact on your health.

Chapter Five

Lifestyle Factors

"The doctor of the future will give no medicine but will interest his patients in the care of the human frame, in diet and in the cause and prevention of disease."

~ Thomas Edison

In hospital-based crisis medicine, keeping the patient alive is the first and foremost goal. In Functional Medicine, however, we are looking at the longer-range plan--3 months, 5 years, and a patient's lifetime. In my office, the personalized treatment plan each patient receives always includes lifestyle modification. Lifestyle skills are comprised of four primary areas:

STRESS

DIET

EXERCISE

SLEEP

These are nothing new but are often the most overlooked parts of treatment, whether you are working on your own, with a wellness coach, or with a physician that focuses on natural treatment methods. Both during and after active treatment, the goal is to have a patient's health controlled as much as possible with lifestyle factors alone.

STRESS

When you think about stress, what comes to mind? For some, it is the demands of work, family issues. For others, it can be fear and worry. Right now, we are in the middle of COVID-19, which has amplified stress for everyone. Many people are working from home, kids are not attending physical school, more people are on the unemployment rolls, and stress levels are running very high for many families. Whatever the stressors are, they need to be held in check. Type the words 'Adrenal Fatigue' in any internet search and there will be hundreds of pages of information. As always, some of it is good and accurate, while other information may be outdated and/or misleading. When stress happens, our hypothalamic pituitary adrenal (HPA) axis adapts to control stress, which is good. The system is designed to ramp up to deal with the stress and then rest and repair. What has happened in our society is that people are not under quick bursts of stress, but continual stress which can cause the adrenal system to wear down. This is seen often when a saliva test is done looking for metabolized cortisol. The abnormal reaction of the HPA system is often the beginning of the downward health spiral.

Think about sitting at a table, getting ready to play a game. You are waiting for the dealer to turn over the next card. The object is to write as many words as possible relating to the word on the card. As the dealer turns the card over, the word written on it is 'Stress.' Most of us are going to quickly write words like work, marriage, finances, kids, pets, weather, traffic, schedule, lack of sleep, etc. That is, most of what will be put down on paper is going to relate to emotional stress. However, there are many types of stress.

Extreme temperatures, for example, are a physical stress to the body that might be easily overlooked. Our adrenal and thyroid glands, along with the sympathetic nervous system, are responsible for how our bodies adapt to temperature extremes. Free cortisol levels elevate more to higher temperatures than colder. It is necessary to gradually increase your exposure to cold and intensity of exercise in the cold weather if you work outside, shovel snow, or participate in winter sports. A surprising result of a recent study.[18] indicates that the hot temperatures of summer are when most people have higher circulating stress hormones.

The interesting thing is that our bodies cannot differentiate the different types of stress. To your body, stress is stress. So, we should treat all stress equally, regardless of its source.

A more commonly identified type of stress is that which is related to emotions. Granted everyone goes through periods of increased emotional stress in their lives but those times should be the exception. Stress is all around us. The question is, are we responding or reacting to those stressors. Emotional stress is a component of every chronic health condition. Clinically, while I am not a psychologist or professional counselor, I have dealt with the emotional component of many thousands of patients. When I talk of stress control, I am referring to the amount of peace and joy that we have or lack thereof.

It is the set of the sails, not the direction of the gale that determines which way you will go.

When I was writing this portion of this book, I was sitting in the shade on the shore of Hanalei Bay on the island of Kauai, Hawaii. There were pristine blue waters, a clear blue sky, moderate trade winds blowing, luscious green mountains to my left, and the relaxing sounds of crashing waves against the rocks about 10 feet in front of where I was sitting. It was one of the most relaxing times I had experienced in a long time. I think about that day as compared to a normal day that most of us experience. Deadlines, tight schedules, news that is anything but uplifting, stressed relationships, etc., etc., etc. Sure, it would be great if we all could regularly sit in an idyllic experience as I described, but this is not reality. Most patients I consult have unrealistic expectations that they have placed on themselves, and often on others as well. How we control our stress determines the level of joy or happiness in our lives.

WE ARE WHAT WE THINK

Our world has become increasingly negative. It seems that our world has lost the definition of tolerance. The Cambridge Dictionary's definition of tolerance is "a willingness to accept behavior and beliefs that are different from your own, although you might not agree with or approve of them".[19] I think that is a great definition. We should all be learning and not have the attitude that our opinions are superior. We need to look at information, think through and analyze it, and then come to a conclusion.

In a recent study titled "Is Belief Superiority Justified by Superior Knowledge?" the research showed that people expressing superiority in their belief claim that they have enhanced knowledge on the issue, however, this is not associated with true knowledge.[20] Across six studies and several political topics, people who were high in belief superiority thought that they knew a great deal about these topics. However, when comparing this perceived knowledge to how much people actually knew, they found that belief-superior people were consistently overestimating their own knowledge. "Whereas more humble participants sometimes even underestimated their knowledge, the belief-superior tended to think they knew a lot more than they actually did," said Michael Hall, a psychology graduate student, and the study's lead author.

In another part of the study, researchers presented participants with news articles about a political topic and asked them to select which ones they would like to read. Half of the articles supported the participants' point of view, whereas the other half challenged their position. Belief-superior people were significantly more likely than their modest peers to choose the information that supported their beliefs. Furthermore, they were aware that they were seeking out biased information. When the researchers asked them what type of articles they had chosen, they readily admitted their bias for articles that supported their own beliefs. "We thought that if belief-superior people showed a tendency to seek out a balanced set of information, they might be able to claim that they arrived at their belief superiority through reasoned, critical thinking about both sides of the issue," Hall said. Instead, researchers found that these individuals strongly preferred information that supported their views, indicating that they were probably missing out on opportunities to improve their knowledge. It's fine to have closely-held opinions, but we must realize that not everyone has to agree with that opinion, and they are not a bad person if they disagree with you. When your opinions start getting too hot, put them in the chiller and enjoy life a little more. We can learn a lot from others who think differently than we do.

> *A fool takes no pleasure in understanding,*
> *but only in expressing his opinion.*
> ~ Proverbs 18:2[21]

In our minds, negativity surpasses positivity. We cannot change events, but we can learn to look at the situation or event differently. Sure, most people wish they would not have to go through the negative events and trials of life, but if we really think about it, these circumstances give us opportunities to grow, develop, and mature.

WE ARE WHAT WE THINK

There is debate regarding the number of thoughts we experience per day. Estimates range between 12,000 – 50,000 thoughts in a day. It is well known that our internal and external dialogue can significantly affect our blood pressure, heart, and modify the biochemistry of individual cells throughout our bodies. A simple example of this is the white coat syndrome.[22] where a person's blood pressure significantly rises when going to see their doctor or even thinking about it. The study revealed that between 15 and 30% of people in a physician's office may be affected by the syndrome. Most of these patients do not have a significant heart issue, but the stress triggers a neuroendocrine cascade effect resulting in altered messages telling the brain to go on high alert. The problem is that, for so many people, this high alert is happening in different parts of the body on a very frequent basis, leading to increasing changes in metabolic function. Outward signs and symptoms can include difficulty losing weight, hormonal changes, poor sleep, anxiety, digestive problems, and the list goes on.

Having seen over 8,000 patients, I am convinced that self-talk can have a profound impact on one's health. Daniel Amen, M.D., one of today's leading psychologists states, "Our overall mind state has a certain tone or flavor based largely on the types of thoughts we think."[23] He goes on to say that, when the limbic system is overactive, a person seems to have a negative filter. (The limbic system is the portion of the brain that controls emotions.) In other words, they focus on self-defeating thoughts. These thoughts severely limit a person's ability to enjoy life and will negatively affect the functioning of other body systems. Here is where the problem for many people comes. Most people who have chronic health issues do not believe they are living life focusing on the negative. I have consulted patients that have histories of some of the most horrendous emotional life histories experiences who have chosen to move on with life and can see the good around them. Sometimes I have wondered how they were ever able to have that outcome, given—for example—the severe sexual and/or physical abuse, not to mention years of emotional neglect they have experienced. I have also seen patients who choose to stay in a negative mindset and refuse to grow. This results in continued health problems, even with protocols that help others with the same problems. I am not talking about saying the right things or giving the right impression. This concept of changing your mindset from negative to positive needs to be the core of who you are. Faking it will not propel your healing but changing how you interpret the negative will allow a more positive healing outcome and change your future course.

Major depression is reported to be one of the most common mental health problems internationally. The World Health Organization estimates that more than 300 million people of all ages suffer from depression[24]. So, why is depression increasing? Brandon Hidaka M.D., Ph.D., cites some of the possible reasons including populations that are increasingly overfed, malnourished, sedentary, sunlight-deficient, sleep-deprived, and socially isolated.[25] I think Dr. Hidaka is on the right path. He is stating that *how* we interact with our environment is the key. This is called epigenetics. Our world is changing, and many people are having a hard time adapting. We are losing our resiliency. Some of the adverse outcomes include a shorter lifespan as well as an increased risk of cardiovascular disease. Faster epigenetic changes are seen in people with depression, including increased aging varied between 8 months to 15 years more than their chronological age.[26]

OUR RESPONSE TO STRESS

Stress is a bigger problem today than it has ever been. One in six children now has a mental health disorder.[27] We are becoming a society that is losing its joy, humor, tolerance, and compassion. I mentioned earlier that as I write this, we are in the middle of the COVID-19 virus pandemic. As a result, daily activities for almost everyone have changed. There is a big debate as to whether face masks should be worn. Let's look at how this alone can affect stress. If you are a mask wearer, you really can't say with certainty that wearing one will prevent virus transmission. You were recommended to wear one and you believed it. You got a mask—not really liking to wear it—but you believe it is the right thing to do, even though you have not seen the hard evidence. The major media flood the airways with opinions about wearing them, but no actual evidence backs up those opinions. When you see someone who is not wearing a mask, it is possible to take it personally. You might think that they don't care about your health or the health of others. So, it is easy to see the person not wearing a mask as a bad person. That resentment you feel for the non-mask wearer is very unhealthy and is possibly making you meaner. It is also making you more afraid because it is a constant reminder that things are not normal, causing you to constantly question the future. So, as you can see, there are many aspects of just this one element of the pandemic that can cause stress.

Everyone has stress in their life. The question is, can you dissipate it quickly, or does it last for long periods? Chronic low-level stress tends to be the most damaging to our bodies. Examples of this would be a long-term abusive relationship, a job that has morphed you into a workaholic, learned behavior of worry, PTSD, and dealing with schedules that are so overpacked that no one could successfully complete the "list" in even a 28-hour day. There is not a day that we don't experience emotional stress. I can't think of anyone for whom stress is not part of their day. Some stress, termed episodic stress, is beneficial. It makes us perform better. Regardless of the source or type of stress we face, in each moment of the day, we have a choice of how we respond. With each choice, there is a positive or negative health outcome.

DIET

Anyone foregoing a proper diet will eventually fall into a chronic health condition. It might only take several months, or it may take many years. The examples are almost limitless, but let's take a quick look at heart disease. It is now estimated by the American Heart Association that almost half (47%) of all Americans have at least one of three risk factors for heart disease.[28] For some, it can be a significant genetic condition, but for the majority, it is a result of years of poor diet, stress, and exercise choices.

I mentioned earlier that my diet growing up was not very wide-ranging. It wasn't until I was first married while attending Michigan

State University, that my wife encouraged me to start diversifying my diet. She grew up eating a wide variety of healthy foods. Honestly, it was hard. She would put a cheese sauce over broccoli to make it more palatable to me, and before long, the broccoli, cauliflower, and so many other foods started tasting very good. I must admit I still don't like cilantro or avocados! The main point, however, is that diversity in your diet is essential. You need many types of vegetables, fruits, protein, and good carbohydrates.

Eating a diet full of empty nutrition (high sugars, high carb) is like driving your car with a tire that has been getting thinner and thinner over the months or years. To drive the car, it seems fine. You have noticed that it does not stop as well as it did, and when accelerating from a stop, the wheels spin a little before they get traction, but for the most part, the car gets you where you want to go. To you, it's not worth dealing with the tire situation when there are so many other things to do and fix. Now you are driving down the highway and at around mile marker 256, the tire blows out, causing you to make an instant decision on how to control the vehicle to the side of the road. The blowout could have happened from hitting a large sharp object at that exact point in the trip, or it could have been the thinned tire finally wearing through. The less tread on the tire, the bigger chance of a blowout. Just like the tire thinning over time with wear, our health declines with the lack of proper food.

Another example would be an iron deficiency. Iron is needed for many metabolic processes in the human body including oxygen transport and DNA synthesis. Iron disorders are some of the most common diseases and can cause a host of different symptoms. Some of the more common conditions include anemia, iron overload, and neurodegenerative conditions. Vegetarians and vegans must be very aware of the amount of iron they take in. The primary sources of heme iron are found in meat, poultry, and fish, whereas non-heme iron is common to cereals, legumes, fruits, and vegetables. The heme iron is more absorbable (15-35%) and other dietary factors have little influence on its absorption. The non-heme iron has a much lower absorption rate (2-20%) and is affected strongly by other food components. Therefore, vegetarians and vegans need to monitor their diet very closely. Approximately 84% of vegetarians eventually return to eating meat due to health reasons.[29]

Your diet is one of the most important aspects of health and it should reflect your metabolic code. Not all of us have the same ability to process the same foods in the same way. I find it interesting that every few months a new diet surfaces, and according to the magazines at the grocery checkouts, each one is the most important and life-changing that there ever was. Apparently, this newest one will transform your life...just like the one before it! These diets are sure to sell countless books, food plans, etc. Aspects of these diets can be effective for many people; however, we must remember that there is no one-size-fits-all when we are talking about nutrition, nor in any area of our health. On the positive side, many of these diets share many of the same recommendations:

- Reduce sugar
- Eliminate refined carbohydrates
- Reduce or eliminate industrial oils

- Eliminate trans fats
- Increase fiber and vegetables
- Focus on food rather than calories

Some of our bodies require higher protein levels and others higher vegetable and fruit levels. Fats got the bad rap in the '70s, '80s, and '90s. Now research is showing that, for many people, fats can be especially important for weight loss, alleviating certain neurological conditions, and athletic performance. The key is to determine the optimal diet for each individual.

Let's look at sweeteners. In the year 1800, the average sugar intake per adult in the U.S. was 3-4 pounds per person. By 2000 that number had risen to a whopping 152 pounds.[30] Unfortunately, many of the other developed countries are not far behind. Between the years 1969 to 2000, cane and beet sugar consumption increased by about 33% and the corn sweeteners increased by 472%.[31]

Top Sugar Loving Nations in The World[32]

Rank	Country	Average Individual Sugar Consumption (in lbs. per year)
1	United States	126.40
2	Germany	102.90
3	Netherlands	102.50
4	Ireland	96.70
5	Australia	95.60
6	Belgium	95.00

7	United Kingdom	93.20
8	Mexico	92.50
9	Finland	91.50
10	Canada	89.10

More recently, we see a trend of artificial sweeteners on the rise. A 2017 report by the Milken School of Public Health at George Washington University shows that Between 1999 and 2012 children's consumption of low-calorie sweeteners (aspartame, sucralose, and saccharin) increased by over 200%.[33] During the same period, adult consumption increased by 54%. More research is showing that the potential side effects of these artificial sweeteners include alteration of the cellular metabolism as well as potential DNA damage.[34] Most people who eat artificial sweeteners think they are doing it to lose weight; the facts sadly tell a different story. This is a significant concern, especially for the youth. The largest consumption of high fructose corn syrup and low-calorie sweeteners is in beverages. High-Intensity Sweeteners (HIS) are a controversial topic, but more data is surfacing each year recommending total avoidance. One recent study looked at the toxicity of the human gut when exposed to artificial sweeteners. When the good bacteria in our gut was exposed to the artificial sweeteners, the cell membrane was damaged.

GLUTEN SENSITIVITY

Gluten is a hugely debated subject with some proponents advising everyone to be gluten-free while others suggest that only those with confirmed Celiac disease should be gluten-free. Again, it depends on each person's genetics. Testing is available to give a clear directive as to whether you should be modifying your diet to exclude gluten. In my practice, almost every patient that has a significant health issue is placed on a gluten-free diet for at least the first month. As they start improving, gluten can be re-introduced for some. People with thyroid, digestive, hormone, and neurodegenerative conditions will most likely be gluten-free for life due to the inflammation it produces affecting other systems of the body. Numerous cross-reactive foods can also cause diet issues for those who are gluten sensitive. Many times, a person will avoid gluten (wheat, rye, barley, spelt) but continue to have health complaints caused by cross-reactive foods such as amaranth, brewers and baker's yeast, buckwheat, casein, corn, cow's milk, egg, hemp, instant coffee, milk chocolate, millet, oats, potato, quinoa, rice, sesame, sorghum, spelt, tapioca, teff, and whey protein.

The reality is anybody can have a sensitivity or allergy to any food causing a wide range of reactions. In this section, I have covered sugar and gluten because they negatively affect more people than any other foods. Dairy is a close number three.

These examples demonstrate that, because of our individuality and genetic variability, eating the correct foods for our metabolism and health now can decrease the risk for genetic coded disease in the future.

EXERCISE

Moderate exercise is essential for optimal health. Physical activity helps keep our organs and brain functioning at a higher rate. People who sit have more issues with their digestive tract than those who are more mobile. One more recent significant concern is the damage being done to individuals' bodies from over-exercising. This includes repetitively running long distances, going to the gym, or other intense activities daily or most days of the week. Constantly pushing your training envelope, exceeding your individual tolerance levels causes performance decline. This is because you are forcing your body to adapt and causing stress on your internal balance. According to the Cleveland Clinic.[35] a long-term excessive endurance exercise may induce pathologic structural remodeling of the heart and large arteries. This is not good news. I have seen more people in the last 10 years have the mindset that more is better when it comes to exercise. They say they feel best when they push their bodies to the limit. Endorphin release is often the cause of this euphoric feeling. The downside is our bodies were not designed for extended this kind of abuse. It's fine to push yourself during an exercise session but not regularly.

Another misconception that has been perpetrated is the belief that exercise is the main factor in weight loss. Realistically, 60-80% of our total energy expenditure is regulated by our basal metabolic rate. This is the internal cellular rate and only around 10-30% for physical activity, which includes exercise.[36] Remember, you eat and keep stress under control for proper weight, and exercise for proper muscle tone. Women especially seem to be under the misconception that they can spend 2 hours a day exercising to try to keep their weight down, only to then overeat—often junk food. When you take the right steps, in the right order, your body will respond.

EFFECTS OF EXCESS EXERCISE

- Excess cortisol (a stress hormone) released causes increased catabolism (the breakdown of tissue)

- Can cause microscopic tears, making your joints and muscles more prone to repetitive stress injuries

- Impact on sleep cycles

- Increases oxidative stress

- Leads to high levels of inflammation

- Increase your risk of cardiovascular disease by up to seven times

SLEEP

We all have those occasional nights that we don't sleep well. Ideally, we should spend about one-third of our lives sleeping. The American Academy of Sleep Medicine reports that insomnia occurs in up to 50% of adults.[37] Sleep is vital for healing, both biologically and psychologically. The normal sleep cycle consists of two different types of sleep:

- Non-REM (quiet sleep)
- REM (Rapid eye movement/dreaming sleep)

Most of us have about 4-5 cycles of non-REM/REM per night. The first stage of non-REM lasts 5-10 minutes. Your eyes are closed, but it is easy to wake up. Your heart rate slows and body temperature drops getting ready for REM sleep.

The second stage of non-REM sleep is also light but produces an increase in brain wave frequency termed sleep spindles after which the brain waves start to slow.

In the third and fourth phases of sleep, your brain starts developing delta waves. It becomes harder to wake up because we are less responsive to outside stimuli. It is harder to wake during these stages, and if you do, you often feel disoriented. These stages are also when your body performs cellular repair, muscle and bone growth, as well as strengthening your immune system.

REM sleep and is the beginning of deep sleep. It often starts about 90 minutes after falling asleep and each REM stage can last up to 60 minutes. This is our dream time, our eyes move quickly in different directions, there is an increase in heart rate and blood pressure. Respiration becomes somewhat erratic and shallow. This phase is important for long term memory consolidation and learning.

The American Academy of Sleep Medicine defines sleep disorders into 11 types.

I find, clinically, that just four types work nicely to stage patients in:

1. **Sleep onset:** Difficultly falling asleep has generally been attributed within the medical profession with psychological or psychiatric causes.[38] With this type of insomnia, it is quite easy over a short period, for it to result in decreased daily activities and impaired cognitive function. I have had patients that are only getting a few hours of sleep and some nights do not sleep at all. All four types can be frustrating; however, this type is at the top of the list. Most everyone has had a time during which they found it difficult to get to sleep. You know how you felt the next day. Now imagine having that problem almost every night!

2. **Sleep maintenance:** Insomnia is the inability to *stay* asleep at night. This can be especially common for women at midlife and the older population.[39] You can go to sleep and then wake up and can't get back to sleep, watching the hours pass. Often people will start reading or use a tablet, which at first seems like a good activity to try to get to sleep, however it can contribute to a chronic sleep problem. The blue screen on tablets, TVs, and phones decreases melatonin, your main sleep hormone. Decreasing melatonin hampers your chances of getting back into a good sleep pattern.

3. **Sleep offset:** When a person consistently wakes early and can't get back to sleep. If they can't, sleep many people think, "I will just get up and start the day." Occasionally, this can be ok, but

on a regular basis, the lack of sleep will catch up and lead to the same frustrated feeling as the other insomnias.

4. **Non-Restorative sleep:** This is when you sleep through the night but wake up tired. You must drag yourself out of bed because although you slept, it feels like you didn't.

Prescription sleep aids might seem to be a good help for these issues. However, in a study published in the *British Medical Journal*, over 34,000 patients were tracked for an average of seven and a half years. The results showed you have twice the risk of dying if you use a prescriptive sleep aid.[40] The researchers also stated caution is strongly advised taking any sleep medication due to the addictive nature of this class of the medication. There is usually an underlying issue that is changing the brain chemistry and affecting your sleep. This can often be corrected naturally by rebalancing the brain chemicals. It is a common treatment that I do. When someone gets a normal sleep pattern back, they feel like a new person.

Key Takeaways.

- The greatest thing we can do is to focus on our lifestyle skills: diet, sleep, exercise, and stress control.

- Stress can be emotional, physical, or chemical.

- We need to be aware of the negativity that abounds around and in us and be willing to address it.

- Eating a diet full of empty nutrition (high sugars, high carb) will lead to progressive disease.

- Almost 50% of Americans have at least one of three risk factors for heart disease.

- Physical activity helps keep our organs and brain functioning at optimal performance.

- A good night's sleep is vital for healing, both biologically and psychologically.

Chapter Six

Four Weeks to a Better You

"Nobody can go back and start a new beginning,
but anyone can start today and make a new ending."
— Maria Robinson

Your health is like a lock. If you scored 0-5 in the FHI, you have identified most of the notches in the key that opens your lock. If you scored in one of the higher categories, you have more notches to identify and fix. My goal for you is to help you find strategies that can fit your life and to share skills to implement the strategies that do not have to restrict your enjoyment of living. We are all genetically different. The only way to have full clarity is to go through the OHA testing for results specifically for you. For some people, the process is as easy as making a few changes and they feel like a new person. However, what I find clinically is that most people need a step-by-step plan based on their individual genetics and require a series of functional tests, as I described earlier. The starting point is the most important part of a plan and this is what has been missed by most of the patients I see.

In the Bible, it says we are fearfully and wonderfully made. I hope that by reading this book, *Intentional Health*, you can see the depth of that statement. Many of you are at the frustration point from all that you have tried in the past with little or no improvement.

I encourage you to put your disappointments of past therapies behind you and take a fresh look at who you want to be. Great health is about adapting to the world around you. By fixing the ability to adapt, you decrease long term illness and improve short term recovery. You can be pain-free, at the right weight, sleeping restfully, with improved memory, full of energy, and have good relationships when you have the right plan. Regaining what you have lost might seem impossible, but when it is taken in small steps, with each step building on the previous, it is achievable. Your biggest decision right now is to determine if you are willing to invest the time, energy, and resources to impact the most important part of your life. Intentional health does not happen automatically, it is a choice. All of this can be summarized by asking if you don't make the necessary changes, where will you be in 5 years?

I hope that by reading this book you can understand why the OHA protocol is necessary to uncover the underlying dysfunction of your health. Since I do not know your specific symptoms, test results, or previous treatment, I will use the concept of guiding principles that will help you move up the health ladder. The following strategies are to start a process of preparing your body for a life of health. For those of you that are already on the journey, simply choose activities to add to your daily and weekly routines. If you are already doing many of these recommendations and are still feeling poorly, I recommend that you contact our office to have the OHA performed because something is being overlooked. To continue doing the thing that is not working for you is a waste of time and energy.

If you start implementing these lifestyle tools, you will likely start feeling significantly better within a few weeks. Within four weeks, you should feel significantly improved. I would like to recommend nutrition supplementation, but I won't because it is so variable depending on each person's underlying problems. Many people reading this book have already been through the "try this or try that" approach. We do not want to use nutrition to just cover symptoms; our goal is fixing the problem.

Let's get started.

EXERCISE

Note: The following exercise discussion is general in nature. Any exercise program should be reviewed with your physician before starting. The following are general statements and do not indicate a prescription.

Exercise is important at any age and with almost every health condition. A high level of overall physical fitness will undeniably allow your body to recover from stress. However, getting patients to embrace exercise as a lifestyle skill, and do exercise regularly is sometimes quite difficult, yet those who incorporate it can have some of the greatest effects.

Benefits include:

- Heart: an increase in good cholesterol (HDL) and reduced triglycerides

- Decreases factors of obesity, blood pressure, and decreases insulin sensitivity to stabilize glucose levels

- Blood flows better, decreases the risk of blood clots, reduces plaquing, and reduces sickness and death

As we have learned, over-exercising is detrimental to our health, but moderate, consistent exercise is essential. Because of our individuality and genetic differences, not every type of exercise is beneficial for everyone. Everyone has a certain tolerance for stress. If you train within those parameters, your body will respond well. Another benefit is that exercise acts as a safety valve for emotional build-up. When you push past the envelope frequently, you will exceed your ability to adapt and start suffering the complications of over-training outlined in Chapter 5. The exception is elite athletes. Their bodies don't experience exercise as a stress event because of their highly trained conditioning. Even when they push past their regular routines, their neuroendocrine system does not sense it as a stressful event.

If you do not have a routine that is working well for you, I recommend the following steps to get into a practice that works for you. If you have been exercising and you feel like you have a good rhythm, keep it up. If this area of your life is not what you would like it to be, now is a great time to start. If you have been trying to get into a program and it feels like drudgery, most likely you are doing activities that are not as suited for you.

Surprisingly, your blood type is a great place to start when planning an exercise routine.

- Blood type A: yoga and Tai Chi to help the ability to cope with stress, reduce cardiovascular risk factors.[41]

- Blood type AB: both intense exercise and calming activities. Use exercise that taxes the cardiovascular and musculoskeletal systems is what you will want to do. Things like lifting weights, running, biking, swimming, and aerobics are good. AB Blood Type persons can handle more intense workouts, and this helps greatly with emotional balance following these more intense activities. Balance with yoga, Tai Chi, or another calming exercise,

- Blood type O: the interval training method is excellent. Let's say you want to start running. You start with a 2-minute warm-up at a nice easy pace, trying to feel as loose as possible. After that warm-up, go as fast as you can for up to 15 seconds (initially, this might be only 10 seconds). Then walk at a regular pace for one and a half minutes. Repeat this 30-90 second split for up to 8 cycles then do a 2-minute cool down. When you can't run fast for the 30 seconds, just walk the remainder of the 8 cycles, or 20 minutes. If you are not strong enough at this time, do what you can with the goal of increasing to more intense activities.

- Blood type B: Balance meditative exercise with moderately intense exercise. Involve other people, with a degree of mental challenge. Activities like hiking, tennis, and cycling.

The recommendation for exercise that I give my patients varies greatly depending on their functional tests. A person who has very low mitochondrial energy might only be exercising three minutes four times a day at only 70% of maximum heart rate because that is all their metabolism can handle at that point. An accomplished tennis player, on the other hand, might have to push to 90% of maximum heart rate during specific training.

10 EXERCISE STRATEGIES FOR IMPROVED ENERGY

1. Check with your doctor before starting an exercise program. There can be underlying problems that need to be addressed before starting.

2. Start slow. It's common for your muscles to hurt for the next few days. If it lasts longer, you are pushing too hard.

3. Your goal is to exercise at least five days a week. Start with every other day to get into a routine then add one day every other week until you reach five days a week.

4. If you feel like you pushed it too much, back off next time. Find what works best and slowly increase.

5. Initially, exercise alone. It is too easy to think you need to keep up with someone else.

6. Keep a chart to see your progress. Often, we have a very unrealistic goal, and it is easy to feel defeated after a few weeks. Break your goals down into manageable units. Track your progress and you will see the improvement.

7. If you can, use a heart rate monitor, such as an activity tracker, a smartwatch, or a chest strap heart monitor. These devices give you constant and more accurate feedback.

8. Make sure to stay hydrated while exercising.

9. Include stretching in your routine; stretching after exercise is usually better than before.

10. Warm-up is necessary. It doesn't have to be long, just enough to prewarm your muscles and joints.

SLEEP

Good sleep is a hallmark of optimal health. Lack of sleep can affect blood pressure, heart rate, mental status, immune resistance, and hormone levels.[42] Chronic health conditions are more likely for adults who get less than seven hours of sleep on a regular basis including depression, diabetes, arthritis, headaches, and asthma. About 30% of the U.S. population gets less than seven hours of sleep, and sleep deprivation has been increasing over the past 20 years. A lack of sleep is most often a result of imbalances in other systems and organs, including hormone imbalance, impaired thyroid (hyper- or hypo-function), blood sugar fluctuations, adrenal insufficiency, digestive dysfunction, and brain chemical imbalance. The OHA protocol works well to get down to the root of many of these problems, but here are some ideas that have helped many of my patients.

10 THINGS TO DO FOR BETTER SLEEP

1. Get to bed by 10 pm every night (weekdays and weekends) with the goal of getting 7-8 hours per night. Going to bed after midnight limits the amount of restful sleep possible, even if you sleep in the next morning.

2. Sleep in a dark, quiet environment, using black-out curtains or shades if necessary. A few hours before bedtime, start turning off some of the lights in your house to prepare your brain for sleep.

3. Our body temperature decreases at night, so sleeping in a cooler room is better.

4. Do not exercise or eat a large meal within a few hours of going to sleep. We want to wind down, not rev up.

5. Do not read, and eliminate screen time (TV, phone, tablet, etc.) during the last hour of the day before sleep. If you wake in the middle of the night, avoid any screen or book time. The bluescreen background decreases melatonin, your sleep hormone.

6. Listen to classical instrumental music with a headset or earbuds for 30 minutes before you go to sleep. Mozart and Vivaldi work very well.

7. Do not watch the clock if you wake up.

8. Some people are sensitive to caffeine while others can sleep just fine after consuming it (due to our genetic caffeine pathways). Caffeine can stay in your system for eight hours or more. Try cutting your afternoon coffee out and see if caffeine is affecting you more than you think.

9. Try to spend some time outside and stay physically active.

10. Avoid using loud alarm clocks. A gentle wake-up process is less stressful.

DIET

It has been said that if your doctor doesn't change your diet, then you need to change your doctor. Modifying your diet is going to be 100% necessary to achieve the goals you want. For some, it will mean some major changes and for others, it will be more minor modifications.

The purpose of eating is to supply our body with the nutrients that it needs. The typical American diet is poor, filled with empty calories, and devoid of core nutrition. 80% of your food should be purchased from the outside aisles of the grocery store. That is typically where you will find the vegetables and fruits, and proteins such as meat, chicken, fish, etc. The average family eats 50% of their meals away from home each week, resulting in inferior nutrition.[43] A comment I hear often is that "Our family is so busy, we don't have time to cook." As much as I understand hectic schedules, I must answer my patients in a manner consistent with what I know and what I have seen in my clinical career. That is, if we want great health, we need to be intentional; it doesn't just happen. The food choices you make can and will affect you and your family, now and in the future. Friends might think you are a little fanatical, but the choice is yours. Do you want to get well, or stay on your present course? When patients start feeling much better and their labs are showing good improvement, I often get the question "when can go to a fast-food drive though". My answer is: "Why would you want to?" My preference is that we would always choose foods that are nutritionally good for our bodies. I tell my patients, "You don't have to do anything I recommend." I give information based on specific testing and current research, as well as provide accountability, but everything is your choice. I am responsible for my health and you are responsible for yours. For people who are put on a gluten-free diet, a minimum of 90 days is necessary before trying to integrate gluten back into their diet. Like all food re-integrations, eat the food twice a day for two days watching for reactions. If a reaction is noticed the food is stopped immediately and not re-introduced again for six months.

CASE STUDY: ED

Ed's wife was a patient, and due to her improved health, she told her husband Ed that he should think about improving his health. Part of his problem was rashes on both hands and face that were present most of the time. The rashes would improve somewhat and then become scaly. The rashes would itch, and he would scratch. As an executive, he didn't like it, but he didn't really want to change. However, he decided to become a patient, and after his testing came back, he agreed to eliminate gluten from his diet. It was hard for him because he would eat out often for business meetings, and he struggled. I saw him a few weeks later with no change and he admitted he cut back a little but was still eating gluten frequently. It was extremely hard for him to consider eliminating bread from his diet. He didn't want others to think he was one of those nutrition wackos. Yet he decided to follow the plan, I saw him every other week for accountability. Within a few appointments, his hands and face were clear. He admitted it had made a big difference and he was getting used to making better food choices when going out to lunch and dinner.

On a follow-up appointment, his hands were red and scaly again. He admitted he'd had a burger with a bun over the weekend after playing golf a few days earlier. He realized how important it was to stay on the diet not just until the symptoms decreased but forever. I think he started to understand it was not just about the outward rash but more about the inflammation it was causing in his gut, which in turn was leading to cell damage. I saw him back a few months later and his skin was doing great. He said it was not that hard once he accepted what he had to do. He did tell me that he tried a few times to go back to some bread, but each time within a day, the rash came back. In addition to his skin improving, he lost 30 pounds with changing nothing other than the gluten.

10 WAYS TO IMPROVE YOUR DIET

1. Eliminate sugar. Help your body learn that it does not need sweets. Occasionally, it might be okay, but on a regular basis, it is aging you faster and creating oxidative stress and cellular toxicity. Foods will start tasting sweeter—too sweet, really—as you withdraw. I have patients that do fine slowly cutting back and others that do best going cold turkey. Craving it is a natural response because sugar is addictive. Eating higher fat foods generally will make the transition easier. No artificial sweeteners.

2. Restrict gluten-containing foods (read the labels). Gluten intolerance or sensitivity is one of the biggest reasons for gut inflammation that I see in my practice. True Celiac disease affects between one and two percent of the population; gluten sensitivity is far more common. When I pull patients off gluten, we see more improvement than with any other diet modification. Remember the foods that can have cross-reactivity listed on page 96.

3. Make vegetables a staple. They are our main source of vitamins and minerals. Three to five servings daily. Eat raw or steamed most of the time.

4. Increase water intake to 50% of your body weight in ounces (e.g. 180-pound person, 90 oz per day). Plain filtered, or reverse osmosis water is best. For most people, drinking that much water is a big change. Start with a minimum of three 8-oz glasses a day minimum, then every 2 days increase by one-half cup. In no time, you will be adapted to your

recommended water volume. Drink half of your water before noon and the majority before supper so you do not wake at night to use the bathroom.

5. No dairy for the first 30 days. It is the second most allergic food for humans. Try almond or cashew milk. Avoid soymilk due to the estrogenic activity.

6. If you become very tired, agitated, or see negative personality traits coming to the surface during the day, eat 6 smaller meals to keep your blood sugar upregulated. Once you heal, you can return to the standard three meals a day.

7. Include protein with every meal. Remember protein does not put weight on; it's the carbohydrates.

8. No soda, fruit juices, sweetened tea, designer waters, or energy drinks.

9. Don't be afraid of good fat. It will not cause you to put on weight and it is particularly good for your brain. A Keto diet that includes a significant amount of dietary fat can be highly effective for weight loss, athletic performance, and for certain neurological conditions. If you are interested, call our office for additional information. Some patients' genetic makeup is more suited for a Ketogenic diet than others. This is another benefit of having your full genome tested.

10. Eat organic vegetables and fruit, free-range eggs, hormone-free grass-fed beef, organic chicken, pastured pork, and wild-caught seafood whenever possible.

STRESS ADAPTATION

Stress modification, like the other adaptations, is based on desire. How much do you want to reach your health goal? If you have been under high stress for a long time, the limbic system of your brain may have undergone significant change and sometimes needs to be emotionally rewired. If you need it, I can suggest programs that work very well. Because we are so routine in life, the stress area can be the most difficult to change. Most of the time, we react instead of responding. Slow down your life and really think about what is going on around you. If you hang around friends that are constantly negative, find new friends. If you are in a toxic relationship, you need to get out. Stress is the silent killer. If you are emotionally weak, you are going to have to learn to say 'No.' If you are a highly controlling person, you will need to find appropriate outlets that are not people. Thinking about what we say before we say it can benefit everyone. We have two ears and one mouth; use your ears twice as much as your mouth.

Having a strong faith is extremely important. It gives structure and meaning to behaviors, value systems, and experiences. Medical researchers have concluded that spirituality is associated with better health outcomes including longer life, better coping skills, and better quality of life even when facing a terminal disease. Depression, anxiety, and suicide rates are lower as well among people with a strong spiritual or faith life.

10 THINGS TO DO FOR STRESS REDUCTION

1. Forgive and be tolerant of others.

2. Look for the good in others.

3. Maintain an active spiritual life.

4. Determine what is important to you and your family and focus on that.

5. Don't live your life trying to impress others.

6. Live within your means.

7. Go outside often if you can; walks in nature are a mood enhancer.

8. Start thinking about yourself as healthy and strong, and that you like/love your life. This can be difficult, especially if you have been under stress for a long time, but it is well worth the effort.

9. Learn to make decisions. Some will be good, some not so good, but you will feel like you are starting to have control of your life. Let no one else control you.

10. Learn something new every day and learn to become resilient.

Professional counseling for unresolved emotional stress can be greatly beneficial if you do not see changes in a reasonable amount of time (8-12 weeks). If you need professional counseling, make sure your therapist focuses on dealing with the underlying emotional issues. Both you and your therapist need to have a defined set of goals to work towards. Taking medication alone is not the path to obtaining a healthy emotional life.

If you do not have a spiritual life and would like some ideas on where to start feel free to contact our office. We would be glad to send you resources.

MAKE YOUR HEALTH A PRIORITY

If one of your major goals is to live a healthy lifestyle, you will need to make it a high priority. When I talk to new patients and go over many of the items in this chapter, the reality hits them that, to change, they will need to act. You can't keep on doing the same things you have been doing and expect positive change to happen. It takes energy, time, and resources. If it were easy, everyone would be extremely healthy. It will most likely be hard, but it will be worth it.

I encourage you to break down your goals and allow enough time to accomplish them. It usually takes four weeks to start to see improvement with chronic conditions. Some of you will notice a change within a few days to a week. It might be increased energy, better digestive function, sleeping longer consistently, and/or longer workouts without pain the next day. It can also be simple activities of daily living like being able to bend over better to talk to your grandchildren or finding it easier to carry the groceries in from the car.

At the end of 30 days, go through the FHI again, and compare your score to your first score. This is a great way to put objectivity to your progress. If you go down 5 points, that is great. It means you are on your way to better health. If, after 30 days, your FHI score is the same or worse, stop what you have tried, and call our office for help. Otherwise, you will only become more frustrated. The same holds true if you start making progress and then hit a plateau. When this happens, your body has done what it can and needs the OHA testing to find out what the underlying metabolic blockages are. This will help you break through to live in great health and get the joy back in your life.

The information in this chapter is designed to get you out of the starting blocks. The OHA protocol is necessary to find out what it will take for you to cross the finish line.

CONCLUSION

I am grateful for the clinical challenges that forced me to dig into the research and develop new protocols for my patients when other doctors gave up and said nothing else could be done.

Every day we all have many choices. With every choice, there is either a positive or negative outcome. The more positive choices you make, the better health you will have in the future. I hope that you achieve a level of vibrant health. I am encouraged about the Functional Health movement and the increasing number of people that have realized conventional medicine will not support getting them to their ideal health. The testing described in this book will help you move forward and get rid of the frustration and time lost because of your weakened health.

I challenge you to start this week doing at least one activity to improve your health. It might be one of the suggestions I have made in this book or it may be an idea from someone else. The important thing is for you to begin improving your health. Getting healthy is not necessarily easy, but the benefits will be well worth it. It is a process of small steps, each one being an integral part of the whole. I think there is no more important return on investment as there is regarding your health.

It is important to get proper functional testing with accurate analysis of the tests associated with your symptoms. Some of my greatest joy comes from seeing once chronically ill people regain their life and say, "I never thought I could feel so good!"

--Dr. Gary

You can always stay in touch at www.goodmedicinefh.com. Links to our social media can also be found there.

ABOUT THE AUTHOR

Dr. Gary Petro is a skilled Functional Medicine physician, with a focus in Genomics, and the founder of Good Medicine Functional Health in Whitefish, MT. He has developed health restoration programs that look at why an individual's health is not functioning optimally, and how to guide patients to solve their health issues.

Dr. Petro has studied under many of the leaders in Functional Medicine and Functional Neurology with a focus on revolutionary microbiome and genetic testing.

He is a member of the International College of Generative Medicine and The Institute for Functional Medicine. Additionally, he has concentrated training in Gastrointestinal dysfunction, Fibromyalgia, Anti-aging Health, Autoimmune Conditions, Hormone Problems, Functional Neurology, Nutrition, Nutrigenomics, and Learning Disabilities.

More than anything, Dr. Petro's compassionate approach to health is displayed with people who are frustrated because of continued poor health. He practiced in Ohio for over three decades, where he directed one of the leading Functional Medicine and Chiropractic clinics, partnering with a wide range of specialists.

He offers secure webcam in addition to in-person consultation for people struggling with their health across the country as well as around the world.

Since relocating to Montana, Dr. Petro is looking forward to learning fly fishing and exploring the great outdoors of Montana. He is an avid skier who also enjoys woodworking. Dr. Petro is happily married to his sweetheart, Mary Claire. He believes each day that the best is yet to come.

Bibliography

[1] McCarthy, J. (2019). *Seven in 10 maintain negative view of U.S. healthcare system.* Retrieved from: https://news.gallup.com/poll/245873/seven-maintain-negative-view-healthcare-system.aspx

[2] Rapaport, L. (2018). *U.S. health spending twice other countries' with worse results.* Retrieved from: https://www.reuters.com/article/us-health-spending/u-s-health-spending-twice-other-countries-with-worse-results-idUSKCN1GP2Y

[3] Ospina, N.S., Phillips, K. A., Rodriguez-Gutierrez, R., Castaneda-Guarderas, A., Gionfriddo, M. R., Branda, M. E., & Montori, V. M. (2019). Eliciting the Patient's Agenda- Secondary Analysis of Recorded Clinical Encounters. *Journal of general internal medicine, 34*(1), 36–40. https://doi.org/10.1007/s11606-018-4540-5

[4] National Council on Aging. (2018). *Healthy Aging Facts.* Retrieved from: https://www.ncoa.org/news/resources-for-reporters/get-the-facts/healthy-aging-facts/

[5] Miller, G. F., Coffield, E., Leroy, Z., & Wallin, R. (2016). Prevalence and Costs of Five Chronic Conditions in Children. *The Journal of School Nursing: the official publication of the National Association of School Nurses, 32*(5), 357–364. https://doi.org/10.1177/1059840516641190

[6] Topol, E. (2014). *PSA Test Is Misused, Unreliable, Says the Antigen's Discoverer.* Retrieved from: https://www.medscape.com/viewarticle/828854

[7] O'Connor, A. (2015). *New York Attorney General Targets Supplements at Major Retailers.* Retrieved from: https://well.blogs.nytimes.com/2015/02/03/new-york-attorney-general-targets-supplements-at-major-retailers/

[8] CRN. (2020). *2019 CRN Consumer Survey on Dietary Supplements.* Retrieved from: https://www.crnusa.org/resources/2019-crn-consumer-survey-dietary-supplements-consumer-intelligence-enhance-business

[9] Biology Dictionary. (2018). *Why Is Homeostasis Important.* Retrieved from: https://biologydictionary.net/why-is-homeostasis-important/

[10] Xie, Y. Bowe B., Yan Y., Xian H., Li T., & Al-Aly Z. (2019). Estimates of all-cause mortality and cause specific mortality associated with proton pump inhibitors among US veterans: cohort study. *BJM, 365*(l1580). doi: 10.1136/bmj.l1580.

[11] Naugler, C. & Ma, I. (2018). More than half of abnormal results from laboratory tests

ordered by family physicians could be false-positive. *Canadian Family Physician*. 202–203.

[12] Genetics Home Resources. (2020). *What are single nucleotide polymorphisms (SNPs)?* Retrieved from: https://ghr.nlm.nih.gov/primer/genomicresearch/snp

[13] Dolinoy, D., Huang, D. & Jirtle, R. (2007). Negative bisphenol A effects on the epigenome blocked by nutritional supplements. *Proc. Natl. Acad. Sci. USA, 104*, 13056–13061.

[14] Gaylord, A., Trasande, L., Kannan, K., Thomas, K. M., Lee, S., Liu, M., & Levine, J. (2020). Persistent organic pollutant exposure and celiac disease: A pilot study. *Environmental research*, 109439. Advance online publication. https://doi.org/10.1016/j.envres.2020.109439

[15] Fleming T.P., Watkins A.J., Velazquez M.A., et al. (2018) Origins of lifetime health around the time of conception: causes and consequences. *Lancet. 391*(10132), 1842–1852. doi:10.1016/S0140-6736(18)30312-X

[16] Mayo Clinic. (2019). *Miscarriage*. Retrieved from: https://www.mayoclinic.org/diseases-conditions/pregnancy-loss-miscarriage/symptoms-causes/syc-20354298

[17] Lindpaintner, K. (2002). Pharmacogenetics and the future of medical practice. *British Journal of Clinical Pharmacology, 54*(2), 221–230. https://doi.org/10.1046/j.1365-2125.2002.01630.x

[18] American Physiological Society. (2018). Stress hormones spike as the temperature rises: Study surprisingly finds higher cortisol levels in summer than in winter. *ScienceDaily*. Retrieved from: www.sciencedaily.com/releases/2018/04/180425131906.

[19] Cambridge Dictionary. (n.d.) Tolerance. Retrieved from: https://dictionary.cambridge.org/dictionary/english/tolerance

[20] Hall, M. (2018). Is belief superiority justified by superior knowledge? *Journal of Experimental Social Psychology, 76*, 290–306.

[21] Crossway Bibles. (2016). *The Holy Bible:* English Standard Version. Good News Publishers.

[22] Franklin, S., Thijs, L., Hansen, T., O'Brien, E. & Staessen, J. (2013). White-Coat Hypertension. *Hypertension, 62*, 982–987. Retrieved from: https://www.ahajournals.org/doi/full/10.1161/hypertensionaha.113.01275

[23] Amen, D. (2008). *Change Your Brain, Change Your Life: The Breakthrough Program for Conquering Anxiety, Depression, Obsessiveness, Anger, and Impulsiveness*. Crown Publishing

Group, 55

[24] UN News. (2018). Some 300 million people suffer from depression. Retrieved from: https://news.un.org/en/story/2017/03/554462-some-300-million-people-suffer-depression-un-warns-ahead-world-health-day

[25] Hidaka, B. H. (2012). Depression as a disease of modernity: explanations for increasing prevalence. *Journal of Affective Disorders, 140*(3), 205–214.

[26] Menke A., & Binder, E. B. (2014). Epigenetic alterations in depression and antidepressant treatment. *Dialogues in Clinical Neuroscience, 16*(3), 395–404.

[27] Rapaport, L. (2019). *One in six U.S. kids have mental health disorders.* Retrieved from: https://www.reuters.com/article/us-health-children-mental-health/one-in-six-u-s-kids-have-mental-health-disorders-idUSKCN1Q02HZ

[28] Fryar, C., Chen, T., & Li, X. (2012). *Prevalence of Uncontrolled Risk Factors for Cardiovascular Disease: United States, 1999–2010.* Retrieved from: https://www.cdc.gov/nchs/data/databriefs/db103.pdf

[29] Leber, J. (2014). *The Vast Majority of Vegetarians and Vegans Eventually Return to Meat. Retrieved* from: https://www.fastcompany.com/3039505/the-vast-majority-of-vegetarians-and-vegans-eventually-return-to-meat

[30] Jensen, H. & Beghin, J. (2005). U.S. Sweetener Consumption Trends and Dietary Guidelines. *Iowa Ag. Review,* Winter 2005, *11*(1). Retrieved from: https://www.card.iastate.edu/iowa_ag_review/winter_05/IAR.pdf

[31] Ibid.

[32] Pariona, A. (2019). *Countries That Eat the Most Sugar.* Retrieved from https://www.worldatlas.com/articles/top-sugar-consuming-nations-in-the-world.html

[33] Science Daily. (2017). *Consumption of low-calorie sweeteners jumps by 200 percent in US children.* Retrieved from: https://www.sciencedaily.com/releases/2017/01/170110101625.htm

[34] Harpaz, D., Yeo, L., Cecchini, F., Koon, T., Kushmaro, A., Tok, A., Marks, R. & Evgeni, E. (2018). Measuring Artificial Sweeteners Toxicity Using a Bioluminescent Bacterial Panel. *Molecules, 23*(10), 2454. Retrieved from: https://www.mdpi.com/1420-3049/23/10/2454/htm

[35] O'Keefe, J., Patil, H., Lavie, C., Magalski, A., Vogel, R. & McCullough, P. (2012). Potential Adverse Cardiovascular Effects from Excessive Endurance Exercise. *Mayo Clinic*

Proceedings, 87(6), 587-595.
Retrieved from: https://www.ncbi.nlm.nih.gov/pmc/articles/PMC3538475

[36] Heydenreich, J., Kayser, B., Schutz, Y., & Melzer, K. (2017). Total Energy Expenditure, Energy Intake, and Body Composition in Endurance Athletes Across the Training Season: A Systematic Review. *Sports Medicine, 3*(1), 8. https://doi.org/10.1186/s40798-017-0076-1

[37] Sateia, M. J., Buysse, D. J., Krystal, A. D., Neubauer, D. N., & Heald, J. L. (2017). Clinical Practice Guideline for the Pharmacologic Treatment of Chronic Insomnia in Adults: An American Academy of Sleep Medicine Clinical Practice Guideline. *Journal of clinical sleep medicine, 13*(2), 307–349. Retrieved from: https://doi.org/10.5664/jcsm.6470

[38] Park, H., Joo, E., & Hong, S. (2009). Sleep onset Insomnia. *J Korean Sleep Resource Society, 6*(2), 74—85. Retrieved from: https://www.e-sm.org/journal/view.php?number=97

[39] Harvard Women's Health Watch. (2010). *Too early to get up, too late to get back to sleep.* Retrieved from: https://www.health.harvard.edu/staying-healthy/too-early-to-get-up-too-late-to-get-back-to-sleep

[40] University of Warwick. (2014). Anti-anxiety drugs, sleeping pills linked to risk of death. Retrieved from: https://www.sciencedaily.com/releases/2014/03/140331130846.htm

[41] D'Adamo, P. (2019). *Blood Group Genetics, Exercise and Stress.* Retrieved from: http://www.dadamo.com/txt/index.pl?1002#

[42] Rasch B. and Born J. (2013). About sleep's role in memory. *Physio Rev., 93*(2), 681-766. doi:1152/physrev.00032.2012

[43] Saskena, M., Okrent, A., Anekwe, T., Cho, C., Dicken, C., Effland, A., Elitzak, H., Guthrie, J., Hamrick, K., Hyman, J., Jo, Y., Lin, B., Mancino, L., McLaughlin, P., Rahkovsky, I., Ralston, K., Smith, T., Stewart H., Todd, J. & Tuttle, C. (2018). *America's Eating Habits: Food Away From Home.* United States Department of Agriculture. Retrieved from: https://www.ers.usda.gov/webdocs/publications/90228/eib-196.pdf